D0149589

Yoga
for People
over Fifty

Suza Norton

WITH PHOTOGRAPHS

The Devin-Adair Company
Old Greenwich

Copyright©1977 by Suza Norton

Permission to reprint material from this book
in any form whatsoever must first be obtained in
writing from the publisher. For information, address
The Devin-Adair Company, 143 Sound Beach Avenue,
Old Greenwich, Conn. 06870

ISBN 0-8159-7404-3
Library of Congress Catalogue Card No. 76-18445

Manufactured in the United States of America

Acknowledgments

I am very grateful to Laurie Jebb for typing the manuscript, Jay Reisinger for running errands, Christopher Wentworth for the photographs, Ida for her encouragement, the teachers at the Institute for Yoga Teacher Education: Felicity, Judith, Mary, Toni, Paul . . . and to Marcia Moore, now in her fiftieth year, herself an author of books on yoga, for graciously consenting to pose for the photographs. I also want to thank my namesake, Florence Norton, for her meticulous editing, her good judgment, and her all round help in making this the book it is.

Table of Contents

Part One

Part Two

Part Three

Looking Back . . .

If I had to live my life over, I'd dare to make more mistakes. Next time I'd relax. I would limber up. I would be sillier than I have been this trip. I would take fewer things seriously. I would take more chances. I would take more trips, climb more mountains, swim more rivers. I would eat more ice cream and less beans. I would perhaps have more actual troubles, but I'd have fewer imaginary ones.

You see, I'm one of those people who have lived seriously and sanely hour after hour, day after day. Oh, I've had my moments, and if I had it to do over again, I'd have more of them. In fact, I'd try to have nothing else. Just moments, one after another, instead of living so many years ahead of each day. I've been one of those persons who never goes anywhere without a thermometer, a hot water bottle, a raincoat, and a parachute. If I had it to do again, I would travel lighter than I have.

If I had to live my life over, I would start barefoot earlier in the spring and stay that way later in fall. I would go to more dances. I would ride more merry-go-rounds. I would pick more daisies.

—Nadine Stair
(age 85)

Louisville, Kentucky

Part One

1

Yoga: Wisdom in All Circumstances

During the first yoga class I ever attended I was situated between two students in their middle sixties. They were bending and stretching like youngsters, while I, not half their age, felt as if my poor, stiff back were stuck in cement. I didn't feel too kindly toward the flexible sixty-year-old teacher who told me outright that "if we grow old and stiff, we have no one to blame but ourselves."

After class I found out that the two impressive students beside me had started yoga just two short years earlier because they wanted to be able to move around without saying "ouch." And now they felt so loose and limber they had every intention of staying that way and no intention of quitting. The sixty-year-old teacher, also a "latecomer," had discovered yoga at the age of fifty, when she was shocked to realize that not only was she "middle-aged" (good grief!), she was *past* middle age! After I reacted with the inevitable "Well, maybe there's hope for me," she told me her story.

"Ten years ago yoga was just mentioned here and there. I must have read something about it in a fashion magazine. What really got me interested was Jess Stearn's book, *Yoga, Youth and Reincarnation,* about how he, a beat-up old sedentary skeptic, started taking yoga from Marcia Moore. The big problem with me was that I had never been allowed to take any form of physical exercise, as I have had diseased lungs since childhood. In high school I had to rest during P.E., which was frustrating because I wanted to play. As a result of having never had any exercise, I never had any muscles. I remember a public health doctor who saw my X-rays calling me up and wanting to know how a person with lungs like mine could stay alive. I always had lots of colds and allergies.

"About the time I discovered yoga I had put my mother and mother-in-law in a rest home. The agony of taking them to a rest home after they were senile made a profound impression on me. I began to consider that perhaps I could hold back or maybe even prevent senility by increasing the flow of blood to my brain through the inverted postures. I think anyone could be motivated by that.

"As I read Jess Stearn's book, I began to realize that yoga would develop me physically *without exhausting* me. Yoga may be done slowly; there need be no strain. I began doing the exercises out of the book. A little later I found a teacher and took my first series of ten lessons, then another ten, and another ten.

"When I first began classes, I came equipped with a giant box of kleenex. Here I was in a yoga class, coughing and sniffing. It was awful to be getting old and have all these junky things happening to me. But little by little things changed. The boxes of kleenex got smaller,

until I was down to just a hanky. Then I was able to do
without the hanky, and I couldn't have been more
pleased. I credited the yoga breathing techniques with
this change.

"I believe it was the practice of yoga that revealed to
me the necessity of taking responsibility for my own life.
I've seen many students able to give up well-established
bad habits with the help of yoga—like smoking, drinking, and overeating. I still have a cocktail now and then,
but yoga enabled me to stop the daily before-and-after
dinner drinks. And that was really a great thing for me.
We do have the choice of whether to live or just exist."

Not long after that, I became acquainted with eighty-six-
year-old Charles, who took up yoga when he was nearing
seventy. At that time he "felt like two boards nailed together." He remembered being so stiff he couldn't bend, and
what was worse, he didn't even *want* to bend. But take up
yoga he did, and he still remembers those initial feelings of
"pleasant agony" as he began to relieve his body of its stiffness and move with an ease he had forgotten. He, too, was
eager to share his story.

"Let me say one thing while we're still alive and happy: Yoga stands out over and above all other forms of
exercise in that it can be performed at any age up to seventy, eighty, ninety, and beyond. Due to the fact that it is
performed *slowly* and in coordination with slow, deep
breathing, it doesn't speed up the heart and is very
soothing and relaxing. The fluidity of the motion of
yoga makes me think of the ocean on a peaceful day
when the waves just roll and roll. . . . Through the
medium of yoga we more or less come to a point where
there is no such thing as time, no such thing as age,
there is just NOW."

When Charles began teaching others, he noted time and time again how his seventy-five-year-old students who *practiced* yoga were in better shape than the thirty-year-old beginners. "I had some young whippersnappers from a nearby university in the same class with some seventy-five-year-olds. These young folks were tired out when the seventy-five-year-olds were still going!" He went on:

> "Animals knew of yoga before man did. Who taught the animals? We can all learn from the way our dogs and cats stretch all during the day. And you can't find a living thing in the world more relaxed than a cat. Did you ever see a cat just lie down and let the rest of the world go by? Now that's relaxation!"

Charles observes that many people find life boring because they have nothing to look forward to. His students, almost all over fifty, and most of them sixty, seventy, and eighty, gain a remarkable improvement in attitude toward life and in their concentration and relaxation. "Lack of incentive makes life dull and dreary. You should have some plan at any age, and mine was yoga," says this eighty-six-year-old yoga enthusiast.

Another student, Marie, in her eighties, recalls how she started taking yoga from Bikram Choudhury. She recalls how she tagged along to a yoga class with her niece and nephew (in their twenties) and sat on the side watching the class doing exercises. She remembers saying to herself, "I bet I could do that if I tried." She tried and found she could. The next day she joined the class. Her teacher was very encouraging, and she kept on coming to class and grew to love it.

> "Yoga truly made a new person of me. I do yoga every morning and sometimes before going to bed. I now know how to breathe properly. What a difference this

makes! I walk two miles a day every day when the weather is pleasant. At one time I had to wear arches in my shoes. I have discarded them because my feet are back to normal. I also got rid of my cataract glasses. I do the eye exercises faithfully. And I had a bad whiplash due to an accident that caused constriction in my neck. For a long time I couldn't turn my head from side to side. Now I'm able to turn it without pain.

"So much has happened to me since I started yoga. Mind you, I *began* in my eighties. My swayback has straightened out. When I exercise on my back, the small of my back touches the floor—that hadn't happened for ages. All I can say is, if only I'd known about yoga years ago. But I learned that it's never too late. Having been a 'Johnny-come-lately'—but better late than never—I'm now a peaceful, contented, happy, and healthy person. . . . "

Meeting these lively people, my stereotyped notions about aging began dropping away. And while this was happening to me I became aware that something dramatic was, and is, happening all over America. People over fifty are waking up to the fact that they are being conned out of the value of the latter part of life by the youth cult. Our whole society is more or less conditioned to the myth that once you reach forty, the road begins to be downhill; by fifty you are well on your way to the bottom; and after sixty it's just a matter of time. Let us look at the facts behind this myth.

Under ordinary sedentary circumstances, the average man or woman past fifty has a substantial sum of unpleasant bodily changes to look forward to. Because these changes are so prevalent in our society, many people think they are a normal part of aging and *expect* them to happen. A few of these changes are:

1. Accumulation of fat, in all the wrong places.
2. Loss of muscle strength.
3. Reduction in motor fitness—balance, flexibility, agility, power, and reaction time.
4. Reduction in work capacity and associated oxygen intake capacity during attempts at hard work or exercise.
5. Reduction in respiratory reserves (breath holding and ventilatory capacity).
6. Increased ligamentous injuries and dislocation strains in shoulders, knees, spine, and inguinal region.
7. Decrease in resiliency and suppleness of the arteries.
8. Loss of calcium or osteoporosis, which leads to a weakened and brittle skeletal system.

The American Medical Association's Committee on Aging, after studying the subject for over ten years, did not find a single physical or mental condition that could be directly attributed to the passage of time. Such alleged diseases of aging as high blood pressure and arthritis are prevalent in the very young as well as the very old. Many of the classic symptoms of old age are the result of little more than inactivity and inadequate nutrition.

The last third of life can be a time of purposefulness and satisfaction. A time to enjoy what had to be missed out on while raising children and making it to the top—or at least struggling to keep from falling to the bottom. These years hold the potential for gaining a clearer perspective on the significance of living. People over fifty who have integrated the practice of yoga into their lives find that it not only gives them more energy to enjoy life, but also facilitates a desire to live more creatively and enthusiastically, literally to be more "alive" than they've ever been before.

2

Hatha Yoga: What It Is, What It Can Do

The young, the old, the extremely aged, even the sick and the infirm obtain perfection in Yoga by constant practice. Success will follow him who practices, not him who practices not. Success in Yoga is not obtained by the mere theoretical reading of sacred texts. Success is not obtained by wearing the dress of a yogi or a recluse, nor by talking about it. Constant practice alone is the secret of success. Verily, there is no doubt of this.

—Hatha Yoga Pradipika
Chapter 1, vs. 64–66

Hatha Yoga is an ancient system of postures, called asanas, flowing movements and rhythmic breathing that help unite the mind, the body, and the breath into a harmonious state of natural health. During the last several thousand years, yoga has developed into a practical, scientific system for enhancing the physical, moral, mental, and spiritual well-being of the individual as a whole. The yoga postures affect every muscle, nerve, and gland in the body.

The science of yoga tells us that our life is not measured by the number of our days, but by the number of our breaths. A harmonious mind corresponds to a slow, deep, and regular respiration; a troubled mind speeds up the breathing rhythm, which then becomes irregular and broken. Yoga teaches proper rhythmic patterns of slow, deep breathing to strengthen the respiratory system and soothe the nervous system.

The practice of yoga increases self-awareness of any disharmonies and imbalances in the body. This increased sensitivity helps us overcome these imbalances through attention to correct posture, breathing, and relaxation while going about our daily activities. This attunement to the needs of the body motivates us to set aside a time for systematic practice in stretching, strengthening, and relaxing appropriate muscles.

As we become reacquainted with that faithful first friend, our body, we revive, bring new life to, deeply buried abilities and capacities otherwise condemned to deterioration and dysfunction. By making the mind and body stronger, more flexible and steady, a person practicing yoga becomes ready to accept an ever increasing responsibility for his life and health and to achieve a greater sense of independence and self-reliance conducive to psychological and spiritual growth.

Yoga is not a religion. Any person of any faith can practice it and find his or her own religion enhanced as a result.

In spite of, or perhaps because of, the vast amount of information in print on the topic, many people still have various misconceptions about what yoga really is. The basic problem stems from the fact that there are several different schools of yoga, each with its own philosophy, yet all striving for the essence of yoga in their own way.

What do the words Hatha Yoga mean? *Ha* means sun and *tha* means moon, referring to positive and negative life forces that are brought together and unified through postures and breathing exercises. Yoga comes from the Sanskrit root *yug* (or *yuj*), which means to yoke, join, or unite. Hatha Yoga is a discipline focusing on the body, intimately aware that the body affects the mind and that the two cannot be divided and viewed as separate entities.

This book offers a holistic approach for the person over fifty wanting to begin yoga in a realistic manner, in terms of the body's capacity. You begin yoga where you are, whether you are a fifty-five-year-old jogger with tight hamstrings, someone tired of struggling to lose weight and disillusioned with "no-struggle" gimmicks, or someone who would like once again to move and breathe freely and experience a good night's sleep.

The people over fifty I teach generally have no desire to mimic the impossible-looking photographs in many yoga books (which is not meant as a criticism of the many fine books on the subject). Many do not even have the desire to become more flexible. But they certainly do not wish to get any stiffer!

The beneficial results of yoga are not somewhere far off in the unattainable future. The body responds with a sigh of relief to the breathing and stretching from the very beginning. But we won't try to fool you into thinking that there will not be initial feelings of "pleasant agony" as you awaken parts of yourself that may have been asleep for years. The goal, if there is any goal at all, is moment-to-moment awareness. Flexibility is not a criterion to begin practicing for. "Real" yoga is not in how strong or flexible you are, but in how aware you are as you experience your body's response in the posture. This is not to say that a goal of loosening up and getting rid of aches and pains has to be denied. In the beginning such goals are what move most of us away from the television set and into a yoga class.

The sense of exhilaration and freedom that comes with the realization of being able to stretch a little further than before, of balancing without falling, of doing things you never thought you'd do again, provides the impetus to keep on with the practice.

You Don't Have to Huff and Puff to Get Results

It is always a pleasant revelation to realize that you don't have to huff and puff to reap the benefits of exercise.

For example, with proper medical supervision yoga can be a wonderful form of exercise for cardiac patients. Studies carried out at Emory University in Atlanta under the direction of cardiologist Charles Gilbert revealed that yoga exercises bring about an improved utilization of oxygen equal to, or slightly better than, that obtained by jogging or running. In addition, blood lactate levels, pulse rates, and blood pressure readings after doing yoga were much lower than readings taken after jogging or running (*Medical World News,* February 1, 1974).

Painful Stiffening Does Not Have to Be Part of the Aging Process

The average person of fifty can no longer touch the floor with his fingertips while his knees are straight. The reason for this restriction of body movement is the progressive shortening of ligaments and tendons. Ligaments are bands or sheets of fibrous tissue connecting two or more bones. Tendons connect muscles to bones. As people grow older their ligaments become shorter and the backbone stiffens. A cause of this shortening of the ligaments and tendons is improper posture and lack of movement.

Improper posture leads to poor respiration as well as backaches, headaches, poor digestion, and other problems. Most people, young and old, use only one-third of their breathing capacity, their upper lungs. This continually inadequate supply of oxygen to the body accelerates the aging process, gradually impairing the functioning of vital organs.

In this book you will learn to breath as nature intended, enlarging lung capacity, consciously expelling old, stale air, and breathing fully and slowly. When you learn to slow down your breathing consciously, there is less wear and tear on the entire body—less work for the heart, lower blood pressure, and a general soothing of body tensions.

Breathing habits are really easier to change than eating habits, but just as important for your health. Any person who has emphysema or who has experienced a discomforting shortness of breath will tell you what a blessing it is to be able to breathe freely. And since most of us tend to hold our breath whenever faced with a situation that brings anxiety, learning to breathe slowly and deeply has the added benefit of calming our minds and helping us to cope with anxiety-producing situations.

It is wise never to jump to conclusions concerning the extent to which a person may or may not be able to restore the normal healthy functioning of his body. When you combine a positive desire for well-being with yoga postures, deep breathing, relaxation, meditation, and prayer plus a natural, vitality-giving diet, you are taking the most potent medicine there is.

3

Yogic Breathing

What is the body if it isn't the soul?
—Walt Whitman

The saying that breath is life is echoed in many languages, as is the concept that breath is the essence, the soul, of man. *Prana* is a Sanskrit term meaning breath, respiration, life, vitality, wind, energy, and strength. Nothing is more vital to life than breath. *Prana* is the source of all energy present in everything on earth—man, plants, animals, sunshine, air, and water.

Once a person realizes that respiration, the breath of life, has a very profound influence on the nervous system, state of mind, and overall health, a continual revelation unfolds. Yogis say that "the body mirrors the breath, the breath mirrors the mind, the mind mirrors the heart, and the heart mirrors the soul, or God." If this is so, then erratic breathing can upset the whole applecart.

To appreciate fully the fact that we have conscious control over the unconscious process of breathing, we have to begin practicing conscious breathing on a regular basis in our daily life. Slow, even, complete breathing is more conducive to a feeling of vitality than almost any other single factor. Many yoga teachers have observed over and over again that older people who know how to breathe well, even those who don't get a lot of exercise or even eat particularly well, are generally in better condition than those with shallow breathing habits.

Through the years slouching in chairs, overeating, work and other tensions prohibit the complete and efficient use of the lungs, allowing the lower portions to stagnate with uncirculated air. (Pneumonia and other diseases of the lungs can often be avoided by proper ventilation of the lung tissues.) Poor breathing causes the muscles of the abdomen, chest, and diaphragm to begin to atrophy. Then, as a person grows older, the improper breathing patterns of a lifetime are a prime contributing cause of forgetfulness, lack of mental clarity, and a feeling of continual physical listlessness. Because we are generally so unaware of this vital functioning of our body, we rarely connect our shallow breathing with the feeling that something is amiss inside.

Complete Yogic Breathing

The process of complete yogic breathing is very different from the usual everyday breathing, in which the abdomen goes in on the inhalation and out on the exhalation. Among other differences, in complete breathing the abdomen slightly *swells* as you *inhale* and slightly *contracts* as you *exhale*. This way of breathing is the natural, efficient method of breathing of infants, primitive people, animals, and almost everyone during deep sleep. If you have a cat or dog, notice how first the lower section of the abdomen swells out and then the upper to complete the breath.

In yogic breathing the lungs are completely filled and emptied as much as is physiologically possible. Complete breathing combines diaphragmatic breathing (belly breathing, common to men) and upper rib cage breathing (common to women who try to hold their stomachs in). Complete breathing offers the greatest use of total lung capacity.

Here are some words that describe the feeling of complete breathing, and it is helpful to keep them in mind as you familiarize yourself with the process: rhythm—relaxation—calmness—gentleness—naturalness.

Allow yourself to smile as you practice. The facial muscles should be soft and relaxed, the neck relaxed, and your shoulders consciously dropped. The eyes may be either open or closed. Opening them helps you to *see* the movement of the body breathing; closing them helps you to *feel* the breath flowing.

Procedure . . .

(Note: Read and reread these directions. You didn't learn to breathe incorrectly in a day. Give yourself time to become familiar with this process.)

1. Begin by sitting as straight as possible in a straight-backed chair, on the edge of a bed or sofa, or on the floor with a small cushion under you, back against the wall if needed to straighten the spine. Or you may lie down, if this is more comfortable for you.
2. Place your fingertips on your abdomen and note how it moves as you normally inhale and exhale—or if it moves at all. Do not interfere with your normal breathing, just calmly watch it and let it be. While you observe the movement or nonmovement of the abdomen, note also the rate of your breath, any quick starts or stops, irregularities, sighs, or whatever (again without interfer-

ing). Next place your fingers on your lower ribs; find out what happens to the ribs as you breathe.

3. Visualize the lungs as two pear-shaped balloons waiting to be filled to capacity, expanding in all directions. The lungs are elastic and expand simultaneously. When you familiarize yourself thoroughly with complete breathing, you will feel the expansion, even in the back.

    (Imagine that as you inhale your lungs will fill with air in the same way you fill a balloon, allowing the breath to flow freely into the bottom of the lungs, the midsection, and then to the upper part of the lungs. As you exhale, visualize the lungs being emptied and expelling as much of the old, stale air as is physiologically possible. But unlike air rushing out of a balloon, you will exhale slowly, evenly.)

4. Now:
    (a) Place the fingers on the lower ribs.
    (b) Exhale the air through your nose.
    (c) Breathe in slowly, evenly, and see how deep down into the abdomen you can feel the air flowing. Then feel the expansion of the entire rib cage. And then the air filling your lungs to capacity, causing you to lift your shoulders slightly (keeping them relaxed).
    (d) As you exhale, relax the chest and release the air slowly, smoothly, evenly through your nostrils. Continue relaxing, expelling the old air slowly from the rib cage. (Feel the ribs moving in.) Now contract the abdominal region gently as you rhythmically expel the last of the old, stale air. (If sitting, be sure you do not slouch as you exhale.)

Do not strain as you familiarize yourself with complete breathing, but do not be lazy either.

When you have followed these instructions, you have inhaled and exhaled completely, thus completing one complete breath (one breathing cycle). Repeat step four several times. Try to make the inhalation and exhalation each of the same time count. Note that as you focus on deepening and lengthening the exhalation, the inhalation naturally deepens.

After you have read, reread, and practiced step four, I suggest that you begin with five such breathing cycles in the morning and evening. When you come to a point where it feels natural and comfortable, then you can focus on making the complete breath *more* complete. *(You may discover that you are already doing what follows next.)*

Remember that since the lungs are like balloons, the back should also move as you breathe. Bring your hands to your waist area, thumbs curling just around the sides of the lower rib cage, fingers spread on the back. As you breathe, feel the back move against the fingers; focus also on breathing *through* the back. Feel the skin of the back stretching as you inhale.

Note: Many people have backs that feel like a cement wall, remaining immobile as they breathe. Many people have initial trouble breathing correctly even after learning the complete breath process because of weak muscles. Continued, persistent, gentle practice will reward them with deep, natural breathing patterns.

Begin and End Your Day with Complete Breathing

As I have suggested, experiment with five cycles at the beginning and end of the day, and whenever you feel the need for a refreshing breath of air. This may take only a few minutes, but it is important that you bring all your awareness to the process. As you integrate the practice into your daily life, you will come to enjoy more and more these moments of "communion with the breath, the source of life." These quiet moments can be a time of real restoration.

After a week or so it is generally suggested that you increase the cycles to ten at a time, at regular intervals during the day, especially upon awakening and going to sleep. As you increase your breathing capacity, never lose sight of keeping the body and breath relaxed, the cycles smooth and even. *Do practice daily even when you miss your asana practice.* In time you will begin to feel very comfortable just sitting or lying quietly for five to fifteen minutes of complete breathing morning and evening of every day, and you will benefit immeasurably from its calming, soothing, and healthful effects.

4

Yoga Breathing Exercises for Persons with Asthma, Emphysema, Angina Pectoris, and Hypertension

> *Every man is the builder of a temple called his body.*
> —Thoreau

Physical therapists have traditionally used breathing exercises to enhance the breathing capacity of individuals suffering from mild as well as severe, respiratory problems. One of the main benefits of such exercises is the increased ability of the lungs to exchange oxygen and carbon dioxide with the bloodstream.[1] Additional mental benefits, such as the lessening of internal stress, have also been shown to be related to deeper breathing. Yoga, with its emphasis on the breath, offers both of these benefits to people over fifty.

The yoga postures can mobilize the thorax, allowing more movement between ribs and sternum, and between ribs and the vertebral column. In addition, the muscles involved in breathing are stretched. The breathing associated with yoga can substantially aid persons suffering from angina pectoris, essential hypertension, emphysema, and asthma. This chapter will deal with these problems and how they are helped through the discipline of yoga.

Factors Influencing Lung Function

Normal lung function can be greatly influenced by a variety of factors. Some of these are physical activity, environmental conditions, smoking, attitude and even ethnic variations.[2] Another influence on lung function, both in the healthy and ill, is the use of a variety of breathing patterns. Yoga uses such respiratory techniques as a central part of asanas, and research has indicated that such training affects many aspects of lung function beneficially.[3]

Yoga Breathing Exercises While Lying On Your Back

Yoga breathing exercises may be of unique value to those with breathing problems for several reasons. First, the breathing is performed, at least in the beginning, while lying on one's back. This allows a greater diffusing capacity for the oxygen entering the lungs.[4] Thus, even if less oxygen is received by the individual, it may be used more effectively. Second, the training serves to prepare the person against future flare-ups of a particular condition that may further restrict full breathing. According to one authority on yogic breathing, W.R. Miles,[5] "Yoga-type respiratory training may have elements in common with adaptation to high altitudes and may serve to fortify the individual against early onset of hypoxia (decrease in oxygen) in emergencies concerned with oxygen supply."

Thus the benefits of living and exercising at high altitudes, which are often insupportable for older people, may become gradually possible under the controlled conditions of yoga practice. Apparently the regular practice of yogic breathing exercises affects respiration by voluntarily stressing the breathing pattern. This produces a substantial reduction in the ventilation volume and in the number of respirations needed.[6] This would allow a person suffering from asthma, for example, to train for future troubles with breathing, and therefore with oxygen reduction in the body, in such a way that this problem would no longer be a strain on the already stressed respiratory system.

Effect On Oxygen Consumption

A third benefit of yogic breathing exercises is their effect on oxygen consumption. Research has shown that the regular practice of yogic breathing *allows a reduction in the oxygen consumption of the person.*[7] The effect appears to be much like that of a trained athletic heart; *at rest, it delivers a sufficient blood supply to the body with fewer beats than does an untrained heart.* Perhaps the ability to consume less oxygen at rest after a period of breath training indicates an increase in the efficiency of the respiratory system; *the individual is actually able to consume less oxygen, but better able to cope physiologically with this reduction. It would certainly be beneficial to the person with emphysema to do just this.*[8]

Emphysema

Emphysema, a disease usually associated with smoking, is characterized by the destruction of the alveoli, the microscopic sacs of air exchange in the lungs. Once destroyed, these sacs cannot be repaired. Although each person has about 300 million alveoli at birth, many of them are destroyed in the course of a normal lifetime by such things as infection and the breathing of polluted air. At the date of this writing, tobacco smoking has been shown to be the greatest single cause of emphysema.

By the destruction of the alveoli, the emphysema victim is always breathless, mainly because he cannot exhale sufficient air for his next inhalation to be full enough. Physical exertion makes matters worse; the body's increased demands on the respiratory system, already stressed just by living, are superstressed by exertion. Exertion to a person with a severe case of emphysema may be something as simple as bending over to tie shoelaces.

Diaphragmatic Breathing

How the respiratory system is so beneficially affected in yoga is related to the actual mechanics of breathing used. Two important aspects of this form of breath control are the so-called glottal breath and the emphasis on diaphragmatic breathing.

The use of lower abdominal or diaphragmatic breathing has the effect of increasing the space used for breathing, thus increasing the amount of air allowed to enter the lungs and the effect of strengthening and increasing the endurance of the diaphragm itself.[9] The mobility of the diaphragm is also increased (a lack of mobility here is common in persons with emphysema).[10] In addition, it should be noted that the pelvic muscles, which support the abdominal organs, likewise affect the movement of the diaphragm.[11] These muscles can be strengthened by the yogic practices.

According to Dr. Mead J. Goldman, "It appears that the diaphragm acting alone is capable of driving the respiratory system with minimal distortion from its relaxed configuration."[12] Thus *the strengthening of diaphragmatic breathing is an important component of overall respiratory health and of the maintenance of that health.* The diaphragm would appear to be the key to respiratory rhythm.

Increasing The Length Of Exhalation

Another emphasis of yoga is on increasing the length of exhalation. This is the glottal breath and is taught to accompany all the yoga postures. It allows the individual to influence considerably the amount of time allocated to exhalation by providing a braking mechanism on the breath.[13] This emphasis on longer exhalation time has proven to be especially beneficial for people with asthma.[14]

Other Benefits Of Yogic Breathing

Other benefits of yogic breathing include the strengthening of accessory respiratory muscles (abdominal, upper chest, and back muscles), the improvement of posture, lung ventilation, and the mobilization of the thorax, the bony cage that houses the lungs and heart. These are all effective in the treatment of persons with bronchitis, cystic fibrosis, asthma, bronchietasis (dilation of the bronchi of the lungs, usually with the secretion of pus), and in pre- and post-operative care of patients, especially those undergoing thoracic or abdominal surgery.[15]

Ironically and unfortunately, "Persons with shortness of breath gradually restrict their activities, and this leads to progressive disability and further decreases their exercise tolerance."[16] A regularly scheduled class in Hatha Yoga, including the breathing exercises, can be a regular discipline to prevent future and progressive disability.

Asthma

The asthmatic too can benefit from learning to prolong exhalation time and from stretching and mobilizing the thoracic muscles.[17] It has been found that asthmatics definitely benefit from breathing slowly. "Less work is required for passing air slowly through the obstructed airways of these persons, as turbulence is then avoided."[18]

Related to asthmatic breathing problems are the psychogenic (arising from the mind) factors associated with this condition. Both endogenous (stimulated by factors within the person) and exogeneous (stimulated from factors outside of the person) asthma have been linked to psychic factors and conditioned reflexes that may play an important role in the actual production of an acute attack.[19,20] *The development of apprehension about the ability to breathe merely serves as a trigger to make the act of breathing that much more difficult.*[21]

Breathing and Relaxation

Most breathing exercises are practiced slowly and should not be continued if or when there is a sense of discomfort or feeling of suffocation.[22] This allows the individual to learn that he can control his own breathing patterns, thereby influencing the effect, both mental and physical, that his disability has over him.

Yoga, in addition to stressing the importance of full respiration, stresses the importance of learning relaxation techniques. *Eventually, the relaxation becomes second nature to the individual, affecting his breathing patterns even when he is no longer conscious of them during specific training.* This training in relaxation helps the asthmatic prepare himself to overcome the panic he may feel during an acute attack.

"Muscle relaxation in the presence of an apparently life-threatening condition is difficult to accomplish, but its advantages are obvious; attacks may be aborted and the quantity of bronchodilators decreased."[23] (Bronchodilators are medications used to open up the respiratory passageways.)

It is suggested that conscious relaxation begin with the feet and gradually move up to the chest; similarly, it begins in the upper limbs with the hands and again moves proximally. (The traditionally used yogic techniques of relaxation are combined with respiratory exercises.)

The Glottal Breath

Another specific aid that yogic breathing can offer the asthmatic is the glottal breath mentioned previously. In this form of breath, exhalation takes place under positive pressure in the lungs. This is caused by partially closing the glottis, the opening at the top of the larynx, or voice box. Normally the glottis, which is controlled by muscles, closes during swallowing in order to prevent food from entering the windpipe and thereby the lungs. When the glottis is voluntarily held partially shut during breathing, especially during exhalation, a pressure builds up in the lungs that allows the escaping air to help force open the contracted bronchioles in the lungs.[24] This process helps overcome the resistance created by the constricted passageways.

According to an article in *Lancet,* a distinguished British medical journal, some people may drift into unnecessary respiratory failure because they do not use their full breathing capacity. The article goes on to suggest that this can be diagnosed by watching the person take a deep breath. It can be treated by insuring that the person continues to breathe fully.[25] Regular and frequent practice of yoga breathing exercises will accomplish this.

Psychological Effects

Besides the preventative physiological effects of such a practice, the entire discipline of Hatha Yoga is concerned with developing a capacity in the individual to maintain a state of psychophysiological poise, even under stressful conditions. Results indicate, for example, that yoga breathing practices help develop such poise, increasing the capacity to withstand the stress produced by the rise in carbon dioxide (CO_2) in the blood.[26] This is one of the first things that happens when a person is in respiratory distress. It also occurs in high altitudes. This double advantage, the enhancement of breathing brought about by the breathing exercises and the accompanying psychological calmness, even under stressful respiratory conditions, are of unique and invaluable aid to anyone suffering from respiratory problems.

Deep Breathing and Hypertension

The slow rhythmical and deep breathing practices of Hatha Yoga have a direct tranquilizing effect upon the individual. This is especially true if blood pressure is used as the index of relaxation. Research in this specific area has shown that results are especially significant in those suffering from elevated blood pressure.

The blood pressure is found to drop one minute after a period of deep respiration. Surprisingly enough, this drop usually lasts for as long as 30 minutes after the discontinuation of deep breathing.[27] It is postulated that this deep breathing may be a concrete way of expressing the degree of psychological tension in the individual.

The advantage of using yogic breathing to influence the hypertensive person can be especially relevant for the elderly, bedridden, and/or especially debilitated individual. A significant effect can be obtained, one that will last. With the use of simple techniques, the person can practice himself, with or without supervision. The techniques can therefore be integrated into daily life.

Angina Pectoris

Another unique and yet little explored benefit of deep breathing is its effect upon acute attacks of angina pectoris. This is a sudden and irregular condition of the heart characterized by severe pain radiating from the heart to the shoulder and down the left arm.

Dr. Aaron Friedell reports eleven cases of angina pectoris in which the patient was relieved of symptoms by the use of *"attentive breathing."*[28] This is the technique that Hatha Yoga has been teaching for centuries. Various explanations for the beneficial effects of deep breathing for angina have been offered. *Whatever the explanation, yogic breathing, with its emphasis on the total slow breath and on the use of the diaphragm, can be of aid to the person suffering from the pains of angina, whether to relieve the acute stage or to prevent and dimish chronic attacks.*

Reduction of Stress Levels

The reduction of stress levels, both physiological and psychological, is related to the type of breathing performed. Evidence has shown that the production of alpha brain waves is associated with a more relaxed state of mind; beta waves are associated with a more active state. In a paper by B. Timmons, and others, breathing patterns are related to the voluntary production of alpha states. It was found by the authors that abdominal breathing patterns predominate during alpha production; beta waves are characterized by thoracic breathing.[29]

This is significant because it strongly suggests that by voluntary deep breathing exercises a person can influence his brain wave pattern, thus signaling an overall reduction in stress levels. Not only is this beneficial during a pathological process because it reduces the total stress on the organism, but it also may be important as a preventative measure against augmenting stress levels that produce headaches, ulcers, essential hypertension, and the myriad of maladies attributed to it in recent literature. This modern assessment of the mental effects of yogic breathing is supported by the ancient yogic literature: "Utmost concentration is invariably demanded in all yogic breathing. . . . It is claimed by yogis that such concentration has, in the long run, a steadying effect on the mind."[30]

Apply These Techniques When You're Healthy Too
The techniques of yoga can be used during health to enhance the normal state of the individual through relaxation training and increased breathing capacity. The yoga asanas can be added to afford increased flexibility and strength to the musculoskeletal system This follow-through approach to health care seems extremely important today when patients are often seen by a string of specialists, no one doctor seeing *the whole person or suggesting real alternatives to lifestyles that may prevent sickness and enhance health.* Such techniques as Hatha Yoga, with its gentle, geared-to-the-individual approach, can help an individual recover his health, can become a part of his daily life, and perhaps can help to prevent further illness.

(Material for this chapter was contributed by Judith H. Lasater, a Registered Physical Therapist in California and a Ph.D. candidate on Yoga Psychology at the California Institute of Asian Studies. She combines her Eastern understanding of the underlying principles of yoga with her Western knowledge of the human body and physical therapy in her teaching of yoga, anatomy, and kinesiology at the Institute for Yoga Teacher Education in San Francisco.)

REFERENCES

1. Brena, Steven, *Yoga and Medicine*. New York, The Julian Press, 1972.

2. Woolcock, A.J., Colman, M.H., Blackburn, C.R., "Factors Affecting Normal Lung Function." *American Review of Respiratory Disease,* 106:692–709, 1971.

3. Udupa, K.N., Singh, R.H., Yadav, R.A., "Certain Studies on Psychological and Biochemical Response to the Practice of Hatha Yoga in Young Normal Volunteers." *Indian Journal of Medical Research,* 61:241, 1973.

4. Knowles, J., *Respiratory Physiology and Its Clinical Application.* Cambridge, Harvard University Press, 1959.

5. Miles, W.R., "Oxygen Consumption During Three Yoga-type Breathing Patterns." *Journal of Applied Physiology,* 19:78, 1964.

6. *Ibid.,* 79.

7. Meduna, L.J., "Carbon Dioxide Therapy." *Indian Journal of Medical Research,* 56:1287, 1968.

8. Personal treatment of private student, 1972.

9. Gilbert, C., Unpublished paper on the aerobic respiratory effects of Hatha Yoga Pranayama compared with traditional exercise. Atlanta, Emory University, 1974.

10. Rossier, P., Buhlmann, A., Wiesinger, K., *Respiration: Physiologic Principles and Their Clinical Applications.* Springfield, Ill., Charles Thomas, 1970.

11. Kuvalayananda, S., and Vinekar, S., *Yogic Therapy: Its Basic Principles and Methods.* Faridabad, India, Government of India Press, 1963.

12. Goldman, M.D., and Mead, J., "Mechanical Interaction between the Diaphragm and Rib Cage." *Journal of Applied Physiology,* 35:204, 1973.

13. Gautier, H., Remmers, J.E., Bartlett, D., "Control of the Duration of Expiration." *Respiration Physiology,* 18:220, 1973.

14. "Physiotherapy for Medical and Surgical Thoracic Conditions." London, Brompton Hospital, 1960.

15. "Physical Adjuncts in the Treatment of Pulmonary Diseases." *American Review of Respiratory Disease,* 97:725, 1968.

16. Woolf, C.R., "A Rehabilitation Program for Improving Exercise Tolerance of Lung Patients with Chronic Lung Disease." *Canadian Medical Association Journal,* 106:1289, 1972.

17. Banszky, L., *The Modern Treatment of Asthma*. Bristol, England, John Wright and Sons, Ltd., 1959.

18. Hedstrand, U., "Optimal Frequency of Breathing in Bronchial Asthma." *Scandinavian Journal of Respiratory Diseases*, 52:220, 1971.

19. Rossier, Buhlmann, Wiesinger, *op. cit.*, 293.

20. Kuvalayanda and Vinekar, *op. cit.*, 52.

21. Cherniack, R.M., *Respiration in Health and Disease*. Philadelphia, W.B. Saunders, 1972.

22. Behanan, K.T., *Yoga, a Scientific Evaluation*. New York, Dover, 1937.

23. "The Respiratory Patient." *Applied Therapy*, 8:30, 1966.

24. Bhole, M.V., and Karambelkar, P.V., "The Significance of Nostrils in Breathing." *Yoga-Mimamsa*, 10:38, 1968.

25. Marshall, M., "Take a Deep Breath." *Lancet*, 1:693, 1973.

26. Karambelkar, P.V., Vinekar, S.L., Bhole, M.V., "Studies on Human Subjects Staying in an Airtight Pit." *Indian Journal of Medical Research*, 56:1134, 1968.

27. Fujii, S., "Tranquilizing Deep Respiration Test in Essential Hypertension." *Journal of the American Geriatrics Society*, 21:153, 1973.

28. Friedell, Aaron, "Automatic Attentive Breathing in Angina Pectoris." *Minnesota Medicine,*, 31:879, 1948.

29. Timmons, B., Salamy, J., Kamiya, J., Girton, D., "Abdominal-Thoracic Respiratory Movements and Levels of Arousal." *Psychological Science*, 27:173, 1972.

30. Behanan, *op. cit.*, 206.

5

Yoga and Back Pain

In finding an appropriate solution for back problems we have again to keep in mind that each part of the body is related to the whole. Backaches may be your predominant complaint on many days, but very likely you also have related disturbances—tension, fatigue, aching legs and feet, headaches, kidney troubles, prostate problems, constipation, possibly arthritis. As you focus on building overall health as well as alleviating the *cause* of your backaches, many different, seemingly unrelated complaints may also disappear.

Chronic backaches should be diagnosed by a physician, since they can be caused by a wide variety of disorders. If the pain is actually related to the back structure, you can generally find a position to alleviate it, such as lying on the floor with your legs up on the wall or practicing the Bridge Pose. (See Chapter 12 on asanas.)

If the pain is caused by a disorder such as a kidney infection, it is generally not possible to find a position that will alleviate it.

Common Causes and Common Sense

1. *Sitting too long* (and consequent lack of movement). Chairs are made to suit an average 5'6" height. The chair you sit in should be just right for your height. Sit in a chair that gives proper back support, put your whole back flat against the chair. Watch that you do not slouch. Foot stools are excellent. When sitting or driving for an extended time, make sure your knees are bent so that your lower back is rested. Check the angle of the car seat for the amount of leg and foot room. Take plenty of stretching breaks when sitting for long periods. After you have been working on your Hatha Yoga exercises awhile and have loosened up your legs and knees, experiment with sitting in a cross-legged position on a firm sofa or on the floor while reading, eating, or engaged in other daily sedentary activities.

2. *Improper lifting and carrying.* Many times we pay no attention to the way we lift and carry things until we feel an unmistakable backache. In lifting, the spine should be kept straight, the knees bent, the weight carried by the arms and then the burden shifted to the legs. If you lift with your back instead of your legs, you are using your spine as a lever. Attempting to lift by bending over puts enormous strain on the back. Don't ever think your back is so strong that "it can take it."

3. *Sleeping in a too soft bed.* Your mattress should be firm, but also adjust to the natural contours of the body. If you already have chronic backaches, it is generally helpful to sleep on your side (relieving lower back strain) with your knees bent. If sleeping on your back, prop a pillow under your knees.

4. *Poor posture.* Caused by one leg being shorter than the

other and especially by high heels. High-heeled shoes throw the spine, pelvis, and posture out of alignment. (For a detailed discussion on posture, see the section in Chapter 12 headed "Mountain Pose.")

5. *Emotional and mental stress.* During times of emotional tension we stiffen our backs. Take time to relax and stretch during such periods. Observe the influence of your day-to-day emotions on your posture. During periods of heavy mental concentration avoid straining your neck or hunching your shoulders.

6. *Weak abdominals* increase the lumbar curve. Strong abdominal muscles are especially conducive to back health. The added strain of an overweight body makes the spine more susceptible to special stresses, as well as making proper posture more difficult.

7. *Imbalanced nutrition.* A diet abundant in minerals and trace elements helps keep the back healthy. Many nutrition-oriented doctors consider a detoxification program (a cleansing diet to eliminate excess wastes from the body) as a primary step in the treatment of backaches. Many nutrients have proven to be helpful in alleviating back pain: vitamin C, manganese, vitamin E. Vitamin C is important in the building of cartilage, collagen, and bones, all vital to a strong back.

(Note: One of the common symptoms of osteoporosis is back pain. There must be a proper balance of phosphorus and calcium in the diet in order to prevent weak and brittle bones in later life. This crippling disease will cause loss of height, "widow's slump," and easily fractured bones. The average American diet of meat, dairy products, and too much sugar and refined carbohydrates contributes to a calcium/phosphorus imbalance in the body, a major cause of weakened bone structure and the resulting backache.)

Yoga and Back Pain

Eighty per cent of all back pain is reported to be traced to muscle weakness or inflexibility. Movement keeps the spine limber and brings nutrients to the discs. When practiced correctly yoga is beneficial to both acute and long-term back problems.

For example, in our directions we emphasize the principle of extending, elongating, and straightening the back before bending. (This principle will become clearer as you practice the asanas.) When practicing abdominal strengthening exercises such as leg lifts and "yoga sit-ups," we focus on minimizing strain on the lower back and maximizing the work of the abdominal muscles. (Yoga "sit-ups" are done with the knees bent, toes stabilized against a wall, going up and down with a rounded back to minimize back strain and maximize strengthening the abdominals. Coordinate movement with breathing, move moderately and with awareness.)

While attending a yoga class never feel you have to do any exercise you feel puts strain on the lower back. Sometimes, despite a teacher's best intentions, the atmosphere seems competitive, and you may be thinking more about keeping up with your neighbor than tuning in to your body. Be careful of this!

Chiropractic

Chiropractic has proven of help in the often dramatic relief it gives to those suffering from back pain and in the lasting correction of many back troubles. Immediate relief may be experienced after a simple manipulation. It is important to emphasize that the chiropractor must be an expert in the field, and reliably recommended. A good chiropractor has to be chosen as carefully as a good medical doctor—and he (or she) is frequently as difficult to find.

The chiropractic profession has much in common with yoga in that it is dedicated to bringing us to a greater realization of the importance of the spine and its relation to many of our disorders. The chiropractor treats not only backaches and dislocations, but a variety of problems that, at first, seem unrelated to the spine: chronic headache, digestive disorders, insomnia, sciatica, among others. Although symptoms of disease may occur in any part of the body, the cause of those symptoms can often be traced to spinal maladjustment.

6

Yoga and Arthritis

If the person who suffers from arthritis is to regain health, the type of care he receives must provide not merely momentary relief from pain, but it must strengthen and rebuild the health of the entire body. One of my yoga teachers originally turned to yoga as therapy for her arthritis, and yoga, together with fasting, nutrition, and a real determination to get well, has brought a lasting recovery of her health.

While generally there is no one-to-one correlation between yogic practices and specific disorders, a well-rounded, holistic program including yoga and nutrition has in many instances brought positive, lasting effects. No claims are made that yoga can "cure" arthritic conditions, but the experiences of people who have turned to yoga and nutrition as therapy for arthritis have shown that by raising the *overall* standard of health of the body, strength and flexibility can be restored.

It is suggested that stretching and relaxing positions, rather than tensing and compressing movements, be emphasized. The gentleness, but effectiveness, of yogic exercises makes them an ideal form of exercise for persons with arthritis.

Many yoga exercises are helpful to people with certain types of arthritis. (Check with your doctor.) Dr. Steven Brena in *Yoga and Medicine* (Julian Press, 1972) explains why:

> All of the bones in the human body are connected one to the other through the articulations (joints). The majority of these work like ball joints. The articulation is exposed to enormous wear and tear because of the dual, constant work it is subjected to during the course of its life. For, besides working as a mechanical joint between two adjoining bones, some articulations are constantly pressed by body weight. Think of the amount of weight the articulations of the lower limbs must support during an obese individual's lifetime.
>
> The rusting of the articulations is called osteoarthritis, and anatomically is characterized by a progressive destruction of the articular cartilages which cover the ends of the bones. When these cartilages gradually disappear, the two extremities of the bones, no longer protected by the articular surfaces, join together, and the whole articulation disappears. If the osteoarthritis—as happens more frequently—destroys the articulation of a hip or knee, one day the individual finds himself in a wheelchair or the dreadful immobility of a bed.

Yoga postures lubricate and exercise these articulations, freeing them from their old "rust" (often calcium deposits). Even young yoga beginners hear cracking sounds when first performing the postures, which in some instances may be the calcium deposits in the joints breaking up (it may also be the ligaments passing over the bones).

People with arthritis should pay utmost attention to the effects of diet on their condition. Many nutrition-oriented physicians have observed that it is rare to find an arthritic person who does not also have problems with constipation (which diet *and* yoga help to alleviate). There are many excellent books on natural therapies for arthritis. Not all natural methods work for everyone—but neither does any other method work for all people. The suggestions for restoring the health of the arthritic person offered in the following books have worked in a high enough number of cases to merit the consideration of anyone with arthritis.

There Is a Cure for Arthritis, by Paavo Airola (Health Plus Publishers, Phoenix, Arizona)

Food Is Your Best Medicine, by Henry Bieler (Random House, New York)

Overcoming Arthritis and Other Rheumatic Diseases, by Max Warmbrand (The Devin-Adair Company, Old Greenwich, Connecticut)

(Dr. Warmbrand was one of America's best-known and best-loved naturopathic physicians and the author of numerous books on natural methods of healing. He outlines in his book on arthritis a program of therapy designed to rebuild the health of the *whole* body rather than one directed only toward relief of the symptoms of the disease. Body cleansing and nutrition form the basis of his approach, together with an understanding of stress, the role of appropriate forms of exercise, and a life in harmony with all aspects of nature.)

7

Yoga and Your Heart

Regulation and Control of the Heart

The heart contracts at an average rate of seventy-two beats per minute. Try clenching and opening your fist alternately at the rate of seventy-two times per minute. See if your muscles don't feel tired after about two minutes. This will give you some clue as to the marvelous efficiency of this organ so marvelously designed by the forces of life. It has actually been shown that the heart runs at approximately 50 per cent efficiency. This is 100 per cent more efficient than the engine in your car.

It is not often that we give attention to our own heartbeat. When we do feel and hear it, it is with a silent, perhaps slightly fearful, sense of amazement. Ancient philosophers and physicians considered the heart as the seat of the emotions. Lack of heartbeat was at one time the criterion for the pronouncement of death, although modern medicine has now thrust us into a shadowland where the moment of certifiable death is increasingly harder to define.

Yoga Asanas Do Not Increase the Work Load of the Heart

Patients who could not be helped by drugs served as subjects in a study of yoga management of ischaemic heart disease. (Ischaemia refers to the condition of insufficient blood and oxygen supply to an organ.) These patients were given yoga treatment for an average of eighteen months. Eleven easy asanas were performed daily while heart rates, blood pressure, and ECG (electrocardiograph) tracings were recorded immediately before and after performance. Deep and harmonious relaxation came between each asana. Asanas included the cobra pose, in which the spine and head arch back while lying on the stomach; half and full locust, in which both the torso, head, and legs arch upward while on the stomach; Savasana (deep relaxation) pose, which consists of lying on one's back and letting go into complete relaxation, as well as other simple leg and arm exercises.

Patients experienced a sense of heightened well-being following yoga practice. Where even a year of usual drug management had not enabled some patients to return to their regular lifestyle, one month of yoga rehabilitated them.

It is important to note that the asanas did not place the patients under stress or increase the work load on their hearts. This was demonstrated by the fact that only slight changes in heart rate, blood pressure, and respiration were observed immediately following the practice of yoga. The postures could then be considered as body building. It is for this reason that the ancient father of yoga, Patanjali, advises doing yoga without effort. (Again, this does not imply a lazy attitude, rather a relaxed, alert attitude.) Economy of energy, harmonizing the breath with movement, and deep relaxation of muscles are essential melodies of the music of yoga discipline.

It was also found that early ambulation of recent myocardial infarct (heart muscle damage) patients was possible. Early ambulation prevents stagnation of blood in the veins and reduces the possibility of thrombosis (blood clot).

(Material for this chapter was taken from *Physiology of Yoga,* by Paul Copeland, who teaches physiology at the Institute for Yoga Teacher Education and is Science Editor of the *Yoga Journal.*)

8

Yoga and Massage

Massage is beneficial for everyone at any age, and it is essential for people who are bedridden or who have trouble with a stiff, painful, or arthritic limb or body. Any kind of gentle rubbing will increase the blood flow and help to ease pain. Gentle touching feels good, is therapeutic, and gives a sense of sharing and caring with another human being.

Massage and yoga can complement and enhance each other in various ways. A massage before yoga relaxes and loosens up the body and lessens the likelihood of strain. A massage during or after the practice of asanas may bring a heightened relaxation and added awareness of the body areas being stretched and aligned. Similarly, the ability to let go into a stretch gained during a yoga session can allow further release and relaxation during massage. Both yoga and massage should be done with a meditative attitude. Both help us to become aware of our energy blockages and energy flow.

Self-massage and massage given by another person can be a part of your yoga practice. Self-massage is often done instinctively immediately after stretching in an asana. For example, loosening and relaxing the knee area with your hand after a knee-bending or cross-legged posture can alleviate any discomfort or cramping in that area. Let your instinct guide you.

In addition, while holding the posture, massage can be applied to the area of stretch to bring both enhanced awareness and relaxation. For example, rubbing the area of roundness in the back during a forward bend can indicate where more extension is needed and also help you to relax deeper into the stretch. Since it is usually distracting to rub your own back (if not impossible) during an intensive forward bend, it is helpful if a person doing yoga with you or someone who happens to be around lends a helping hand. Massage after or before deep yoga relaxation is especially rewarding if the session has been very intense.

(For a more thorough discussion about "instinct-directed" self-massage, see *The First Book of Do-In,* by Jacques de Langre, published by Happiness Press, Magalia, California 95954.)

Touch Is Healing

Delores Krieger, a registered nurse at New York University, has been conducting experiments showing that the touch of a "psychic healer" causes the hemoglobin level in the blood to rise. Under carefully controlled conditions she tested the blood of seriously ill patients both before and after they were exposed to the "laying on of hands" from a professed spiritual healer. She believes that the hemoglobin increase is a significant physiological indication that the healing process is actually taking place. Through her extensive work with "touch" healing she finds she has picked up the ability herself and concludes that the technique is eminently teachable. Sister Justa M. Smith, a

Buffalo, N.Y., biochemist, was the discoverer of this hemo-globin response to "healing hands."

Foot Massage

Before this modern era of cement, hard shoes, and floors people had more opportunity to go barefoot in a natural environment, stepping on stones and sticks, which pressed into the "reflexes" on the bottoms of their feet. This natural foot massage helped keep the various nerve endings in the feet free from congestion and stimulated normal circulation to every part of the body.

The less we walk freely on grass, sand, leaves, dirt, and pebbles, the more we can benefit from an exceedingly sim-ple method of foot massage generally referred to as foot reflexology.

There are several informative books written on "helping yourself with reflexology"—though admittedly, at first glance, some of the reflex point charts look a little compli-cated. However, unless you want to work on a specific ail-ment, you don't have to know all the exact points; just go over the whole foot.

A foot massage is pleasant to give to a friend and a plea-sure to receive. It can be a fun ice-breaker at a social get-together—and a lot better for everyone than that extra cocktail. Any number of people can form a circle to give and receive a foot massage at the same time. A group of three or four people working on each other's feet even helps to stimulate spontaneous, nonmonotonous conversa-tion. Don't worry about exactly how to do it. Pretend you are doing your *own* feet and just let the warmth and good energy flow through your hands.

Some people claim that standing in a shoe box full of marbles feels great, or they roll their feet on a soda pop bottle. Others use foot massage sandals or a device on the market called a "Reflex Massager." Find a way to incorporate foot massage in your own routine. Especially on days when you cannot spend time barefoot outdoors, take a few minutes after your yoga practice to do the following:

1. Gently twist and squeeze each toe.
2. Spread the toes apart and massage between them.
3. Press your fingers at the connection of the toes and top of the foot.
4. Knead the foot with your thumbs, massaging sensitive areas with a gentle, circular motion.
5. Make a fist and press your knuckles down on the outside of the foot; move down from the toe to the heel firmly three times, and from the center of the foot to the heel three times.
6. Slap the foot gently with the palm and once again, for good measure, firmly rub the entire sole.
7. Be sure to do both feet!

For strengthening the feet and making the toes flexible, practice picking up cloth or marbles with the toes. Pick your socks up with your toes!

If you are interested in pursuing the subject further, the following books will be helpful:

Stories the Feet Can Tell (paper $2.50; cloth $3.50)
Stories the Feet Have Told (paper $3.95; cloth $4.50)
   (Both available by writing to P.O. Box 948, Rochester, N.Y. 14603)
Helping Yourself with Foot Reflexology, by Mildred Carter ($2.45)
   (Parker Publishing Company, c/o Prentice-Hall, Inc., Englewood Cliffs, N.J. 07632)

Dry Brush Massage

Dry brush massage is an easy, convenient way of revitalizing the skin and increasing its capacity to eliminate waste products. You need a suitable brush, preferably a natural bristle brush about the size of your hand or larger, with a long handle so you can reach down your back. Or use either a regular, inexpensive natural-plant fiber vegetable brush, a coarse bath glove, or a "loofah mitt," which is a coarse, natural sponge. Do not use nylon or synthetic brushes, as these will damage your skin. You can of course "wet-brush" massage yourself while in the bath or shower, but "dry-brush" massaging is more effective for some people.

It is advisable to start out with a less harsh brush and brush gently at first. Start with the soles of your feet, brush in a rotary motion, then the legs, hands, arms, back, abdomen, chest, and neck. Brush until your skin becomes rosy, warm, and glowing, about five minutes. Remember, start out gently, moderately. If done regularly, dry-brush massage will

1. Remove dead layers of skin and other impurities, keep the pores open.
2. Stimulate and increase blood circulation in all underlying organs and tissues.
3. Increase the eliminative capacity of your skin.
4. Stimulate the hormone- and oil-producing glands.
5. Stimulate nerve endings in the skin.
6. Help prevent colds, especially when followed by a cool shower.
7. Make your skin look fresher.
8. Improve your health generally and help you become aware that your skin is a living, vital organ.

9

Relaxing Your Way to Better Health

A merry heart doeth good like a medicine:
but a broken spirit drieth the bones.
—Proverbs 17:22

It has been estimated that three out of every four visits to the family doctor in the U.S. today are for psychosomatic or stress-related problems, and that valium, a tranquilizer, is one of the most commonly prescribed drugs. As the effects of yoga become more understood by the medical community, yoga and yoga-related practices (such as bio-feedback) will very likely become routinely recommended for everyone.

As people who suffer from them know, psychosomatic illnesses are *not* "all in your head." Experiments have shown that every emotion automatically produces certain physical changes in the body. Stress (defined as wear and tear on the body, brought about by any activity) can be produced by feelings and emotions. Paul Copeland, author of *Physiology of Yoga,* explains it this way:

Whenever you are in a situation of threat, your body prepares to fight or flee. In a moment of peril everything gets into the act. First, messages from your eyes and ears get relayed, via the cerebral cortex and other brain structures, to the pituitary gland at the base of the brain. A substance known as ACTH is released and goes to stimulate the adrenal glands atop the kidneys. These then secrete a class of hormones known collectively as the glucocorticoids. They assist the body in the necessary mobilization of stored energy. In addition, the brain sends messages directly to other body organs via the autonomic nervous system to increase heart rate, change blood flow and other functions. You are now prepared to cope with the stress.

If the provocation is minor—if it's not necessary to fight—then the body undergoes this stress for no good reason. You can't punch a mechanic in the nose because he charged you a hundred dollars and didn't fix the carburetor, so you suffer quietly while your stomach ulcerates.

Through the years major tensions may accumulate and bring maladjustments between organs of the body, which may in turn affect our thinking. When the body is repeatedly battered with negative emotions, it breaks down at its weakest point, and illness results. The list of diseases thought to be initiated by our emotions is almost endless.

Positive feelings, on the other hand, bring new life to the body. Dr. Hans Selye, Director of the Institute of Experimental Medicine and Surgery at the University of Montreal and author of a number of books on stress, has stated in *Stress Without Distress* (J.B. Lippincott Company):

There exists a close relationship between work, stress and aging. Aging results from the sum of all the stresses to which the body has been exposed during a lifetime. Each period of stress—especially if it derives from frustrating, unsuccessful struggles—leaves some irreversible chemical scars, which accumulate to constitute the signs of tissue aging. But successful activity, no matter how intense, leaves you with comparatively few such scars. On the contrary, it provides you with the exhilarating feeling of youthful strength, even at a very advanced age. Work wears you out mainly through the frustration of failure. Many of the eminent among the hard workers in almost any field have lived a long life . . . well into their seventies, eighties or even late nineties. They lived . . . a life of constant leisure by always doing what they like to do.

It is true that few people belong to this category of the creative elite; admittedly their success in meeting the challenge of stress cannot serve as a basis for a general code of behavior. But you can live long and happily by working hard along more modest lines if you have found the proper job and are reasonably successful at it.

Biofeedback

We are learning that people have a lot more control over the way their bodies function than was previously thought possible. In addition to mind/body practices such as Hatha Yoga, the link between mind and body has been intensively explored in a new field of study called biofeedback. Biofeedback is essentially a particular kind of feedback—feedback from different parts of our body: the brain, the heart, the circulatory system, the different muscle groups, and so on. Biofeedback training teaches a person to tune in to his bodily functions and eventually to control them.

In case you have managed to miss the numerous books and news articles on biofeedback, it works basically as follows: In a typical training session a person is exposed to his feedback by hooking up with equipment that can amplify one or more of his body signals and translate them into easily observable signals, such as a flashing light, the movement of a needle, a steady tone, or the squiggle of a pen. Once a person can "see" his heartbeats or "hear" his brain waves he has the information needed to begin to learn controlling them. People have taught themselves to lower their blood pressure, increase poor circulation to their extremities, prevent migraine headaches, and overcome insomnia through biofeedback training.

There are many activities conducive to relaxation—a walk along the beach or in a beautiful park, a hike in the mountains, drawing, music, gardening, a sport you enjoy, even cooking for some. We need to listen when our body tells us to partake of them. Sometimes we come to a point in our life when we approach everything with tension and apprehension, when even activities that were once relaxing fail to relax us. In fact, this tension becomes so much a part of us we no longer notice it. The yoga asanas, the attention to breathing patterns, and learning to relax the body consciously offer a pause between habitually uptight activities. This pause can serve as a contrast for the tense person and help to break up a vicious circle, as well as retraining both mind and body to relax voluntarily.

Mantra

It is possible to slow your pulse and breathing, lower your blood pressure, and calm your mind simply by sitting still and concentrating on a ticking clock or dripping faucet. Scientific tests have shown that repetition of any words or sounds (hummmm . . . ommmm . . . laaaaa . . .) are, at least from a physical point of view, as useful as a "mantra."

A mantra is considered to be a syllable, word, name, phrase, or sound that derives its effectiveness by attuning the vibration of the individual to the "cosmic" through sound. A true mantra is said to carry the potential of bringing the seeker to the goal of total inner freedom. Some "spiritual" teachers say that mantra repetition makes the mind dull and mechanical, that it is something to pacify gullible people. Other teachers praise it.

Some say that a true mantra cannot be fabricated out of midair, although the experiments of Dr. Herbert Benson (author of *The Relaxation Response,* William Morrow Company) indicate that any word will do. Dr. Benson, using the word "one" like a mantra, apparently achieved psychological results similar to those claimed for so-called "Transcendental Meditation." (By definition, any activity that helps us transcend the hubbub of daily life is "transcendental.")

I leave it to you to discover for yourself, if you wish, whether repetition of a mantra is an aid to "spiritual" awakening. Let us say simply that a mantra or word, combined with breathing, has the potential of focusing your mental and emotional energies. There are times when this can be a valuable practice.

OM or AUM

Om or Aum, as it is sometimes written, is a pleasant, soothing, familiar sound and generally easily chanted without a feeling of self-consciousness.

How to form the sound of Om: Lying down or sitting up, inhale deeply, and on the exhalation sound "Oooo." (pronounced as in "oh"), abruptly switch to "mmmmm" (equal length to the "ooooo"), continuing until the lungs are almost empty. The sound should be made as evenly as possible; sometimes it will feel right to sound it forcefully, sometimes softly.

Other Sounds

The effect of sound is said to change with every vowel. Different sounds are said to be helpful in cleansing and recharging our system.

The sound "ee" (as in "bee") is said to affect the pituitary and pineal glands, the brain and all the other organs in the head. The sound "ea" (as in "heavy") affects the thyroid and parathyroid, the trachea, the larynx, and the throat. The sound "ah" (as in "awesome") affects the upper part of the lungs. The sound "oh" (as in "Rome") affects their lower part. The sound "oo" (as in "broom") affects the lower organs and sex glands. All the organs situated in the area of the lungs, including the heart, are benefited by the "ah" and "oh" sounds. The sound "ohm" is said to affect the heart particularly. (These vowels are chanted on an exhalation.)

First, as with "ohm," inhale deeply, then chant the vowel with the full force of the exhaling breath, shaping your mouth according to the vowel. In "ee" the lips are in a slight smile, in "ah" the mouth is wide open, in "oh" the lips are pursed, and in "oo" they are puckered up as if starting to whistle.

Make a clear, strong tone. Do each sound three or four times, trying to visualize the sound and the related part of the body. These vibrations are pleasant. Explore their possibilities with an open mind.

10

Sleep

Sleep that knits up the ravell'd sleave of care,
The death of each day's life, sore labour's bath,
Balm of hurt minds, great nature's second course,
Chief nourisher in life's feast.
—Shakespeare

Beginnings and endings—life is full of them. Our days begin when we wake up and end when we fall asleep. And what goes on in that mysterious in-between transition state? There are as many speculations about sleep as there are about death, and in some ways sleep is like a gentle death.

While our understanding of sleep is far from complete, it is clear that what restores our energies is not the amount of sleep, but the quality. Unfortunately, many of us have become so accustomed to filling up our time with busy activities that we leave this one-third of our life to chance. The fact that this society takes billions of dollars of sedatives, tranquilizers, and awakeners is an indication that the way we live our lives during the day is not conducive to a good night's rest.

The body is a most sensitive, intricate instrument. Studies have shown that drug-induced sleep is not the same as normal sleep. Many natural stages and rhythms are upset, and activity in the areas of the brain considered responsible for integrating experience is hindered.

There are many ways to prepare for peaceful, restful sleep. The practice of asanas and breathing cycles before going to sleep is conducive to clearing the mind, to letting go of the past day's events and the next day's expectations. Asanas relax the body so that we don't plop into bed in a state of bottled tension that results in tossing and turning through the night. It is unrealistic to expect to sleep peacefully when your mind is full of last-minute impressions from a late television show or an exciting book or business worries. Continuing with stimulating activities until you feel too tired to go on can result in a drained feeling when you are finally in bed; you may long for peaceful oblivion, but the mind just won't turn off.

Overeating and drinking too close to bedtime is usually asking for trouble. And if you watch television and eat at the same time, you are *really* asking for trouble. Nature is a wise mother who must be listened to. Eating long after sunset or engaging in too many activities in artificial light are not consistent with her natural rhythms.

At least an hour before bedtime stay away from activities that set your mind spinning and make you feel keyed up inside. Evening activities you really enjoy should be sought out, but don't let social pressure or the desire to "stay with it" exhaust you to the point where you can't get to sleep.

If you are worried or find yourself planning something as you try to doze off, it sometimes helps to turn on the night light or even to light a candle (bright light may stimulate you too much) and scribble your thoughts on a piece of paper.

Other Miscellaneous Considerations To Improve Sleep

1. Stepping outside and breathing in the cool night air, taking in the vastness and beauty of the heavens, helps to put one's concerns in perspective.
2. Sleep in quiet, dark surroundings.
3. A cup of warm camomile tea taken an hour before bedtime is relaxing and also helps relieve excess gas in the system. Other helpful herb teas for insomnia include licorice root, chaparral, valerian, and hops.
4. A warm bath.
5. Rest your feet in cool water. Dry briskly with a rough towel. Then apply some oil (not mineral) to each foot. Massage the feet while consciously letting go of the thoughts of the day as they come up, allowing the mind to be clear and carefree. Don't take your worries to bed with you. Give particular attention to massaging the areas of the foot in the arch and the pads between the toes.
6. Listen to soothing music.
7. Chant Om (Ohm) silently or aloud.
8. Relax in Child's or Hare Pose. (See Chapter 12 on asanas.) Rest on slant board.
9. The mattress you sleep on should be firm, not soft and saggy, if you want to avoid backaches and treat your spine to good health.
10. The room should be well ventilated, neither too cold nor too stuffy.
11. Practice deep breathing in bed with the fingertips on the solar plexus. The rhythmical rise and fall of the stomach has a soothing effect, taking gentle deep breaths as you practice deep relaxation by exhaling tension from

each part of your body. You cannot force your body to sleep; you can allow it to fall asleep by being relaxed and receptive to sleep.

12. If all else fails, try this: Get out of bed, put your yoga pad on the floor, a blanket on top of the pad if necessary, and some blankets beside the pad. Turn on a dim night light. Relax on your back on the pad and practice a few yoga positions, such as the Bridge Pose, the Knee to Chest Pose, or whatever other movements on the back you may feel like doing. Then, if you still don't feel really drowsy resting between the poses, sit up on the pad and work very lazily on the forward bends, taking care to relax into each stretch. Then lie down again, cover yourself with the blankets, put a small pillow under your head if you like, and practice deep relaxation. If you feel yourself starting to fade away, you can either stumble back to bed or just go to sleep where you are. (You can, of course, do the asanas in bed, but leaving the bed takes away the pressure of *having* to fall asleep.)

And Upon Awakening . . .

Let's hope you are not being awakened by an alarm or have to panic, rush, and immediately jump out of bed when you've overslept half an hour. Some of us habitually jump out of bed upon awakening, others bury themselves deeper under the covers, try to sneak a few more winks, and then jump out of bed anyway at the last minute.

Before we consciously awaken in the morning the mind gives a "signal" that it's time to wake up. It is far healthier for your nervous system and much more energizing if you awaken gradually and consciously, even if this involves having to wake up fifteen minutes earlier.

First, take time to learn about yourself. What waking-up habits have you fallen into over the past fifty, sixty, seventy, or eighty years? The start of the day is as important as its finish. Maybe there is little that needs changing, and maybe you will discover that there are better ways to awaken.

When first coming out of sleep, lie quietly with your eyes closed and give attention to what your mind and body feel like. Listen to the sounds, and the silence between the sounds, all around you. Then, when you feel ready, slowly open your eyes. What is it like to see the world for the very first time? Allow your eyes to feel soft, and soften the gaze. Whether you are nearsighted, farsighted, or have 20/20 vision, see if you can tune into allowing your vision to come *to* you. Continue to lie peacefully in bed a little longer as you experience the beginnings of waking.

Then, if you don't yawn naturally, begin to yawn deliberately. At the same time, slowly, leisurely, naturally, begin to stretch your arms, hands, fingers, legs, feet, and toes. Slowly turn and twist and stretch all over your body. Stretch your arms and legs slowly, several times. Turn and twist your body from your pelvis to your neck. Open and close your hands and fingers. Wiggle your toes. And as you leisurely stretch all over, take soft, easy, gentle, deep breaths.

Continue to inhale, exhale, yawn, yawn, and begin to smile and allow the jaw to feel loose and relaxed. Direct your thoughts to being positive. Know that you are going to be kind and good to yourself today, that this day you are not starting out with your body "uptight," but that you are going to allow your body to feel as comfortable and supple as possible.

PART TWO

11

The Learning and Practice of Yoga

Yoga Classes

It is possible to learn yoga from a book, just as it is possible to take a "learn-to-draw-in-six-easy-lessons" correspondence course. But the instructions in a book will hopefully make more sense after having seen the asanas demonstrated by a teacher.

Today yoga classes are sponsored through adult education programs, health clubs, women's clubs, centers for senior citizens, churches, synagogues, YMCA's and YWCA's, yoga institutes and as part of recreational and school programs. You can go to yoga retreats and resorts teaching yoga, or you can find yoga teachers with classes in their homes or studios. If a class is not available in your area, you can probably get a class going by calling a nearby yoga organization or yoga teachers' training program and helping to arrange for the use of a room (through your church, for example) in which the class can be conducted. The classes I first taught for people over sixty were held in a spare room at a lovely teachers' retirement home. If you have several friends desiring to take up yoga, perhaps you can move the furniture back in the living room and get a teacher to come to your home.

There are many different approaches to the teaching of yoga, as people who have gone "yoga teacher shopping" know. At one point, when I first began learning yoga, I was attending the classes of five different teachers, and it seemed that they each had a slightly different way of doing essentially the same pose; many times they even called the same pose by a different name. Some of these classes were held by candlelight, the teacher speaking very softly and telling the students to "just relax . . .relax . . . relax." Others were held in well-lit rooms, the teacher not only speaking in a normal tone, but even raising his voice in slight frustration as he urged us to "try a little harder . . . stretch a little further . . . hold a little longer." I could see advantages and disadvantages to each approach.

Sooner or later the student who practices at home as well as in class discovers that "the teacher instructs, but the body teaches." Never follow any teacher blindly. Teachers are also still students and consequently always learning and changing. It's great if you can find a teacher who seems to be on the same wavelength as you are, but even if you don't feel immediate rapport, you can learn just the same as long as the teacher's instructions are clear.

For you to get the most out of a class the teacher must have the time and capacity to focus on you as an individual, giving encouragement and help where it is needed. Group lessons are fun, especially with people you know or can get acquainted with. But the class should not contain more students than the teacher can supervise and give individual attention to as needed. It should not be so crowded that you have to strain your eyes and ears to find out what the teacher is demonstrating.

Beginners of any age generally feel at ease in a class of people with similar abilities, where they will be able to participate in the entire session. There are excellent classes with the postures done sitting in a chair or standing up. Take time to find out what type of group situation is best for you. Some yoga teachers believe in seeing new students on an individual basis to find out what sort of group program is most appropriate for them and which particular postures would be most helpful. Private lessons are more expensive, but they are priceless if you find a knowledgeable teacher who may be able to instruct you in the postures most suited to your specific needs.

A preregistered series of six to ten lessons is usually best for both student and teacher. If you miss a class or two, you may feel awkward about coming back, especially if the rest of the class has made progress. If you are truly sincere about learning yoga, most teachers will be very understanding and happy to see you back. For many teachers it hasn't been very long since they too were trying to establish a yoga routine in their own life, and they remember well their own difficulties in getting started.

At-Home Routine

The suggestions below will take on different meanings as you progress in your practice and become increasingly familiar with your body's response to the postures.

The Eyes

In the beginning I suggest that you keep your eyes open, even after you have learned the technique by reading and rereading the instructions and by attending a yoga class. (Hopefully you will have the opportunity to do both.) When your eyes are open, you can check your body alignment and make the necessary corrections. Some yoga teachers suggest closing the eyes from the very beginning to help remove outside distractions and to experience more fully what is happening to the body. After you become acquainted with the technique of doing a particular asana, you might try moving into it with your eyes open, holding it motionless with your eyes closed, and coming out of it with your eyes either open or closed.

How to Practice the Asanas

Common sense is your ultimate guide. You move into a pose slowly, with awareness, and pause at the point of "feeling it." At that point, you remain as motionless as possible and experience your body's response to the asana with as little resistance as possible. If you feel able, before releasing the motionless hold, see if you can stretch a little further as you exhale. Save enough energy to come out of the pose with awareness. In other words, never hold to the point where you collapse.

Rest between each pose, about the same amount of time as you held the pose, but not so long that you lose the feeling of being "warmed up." It is often beneficial to repeat a pose two or three times. Allow the breath and pulse rate to return to normal before you practice the next asana.

Be sure not to hold your breath during a posture! With practice the movement and the breath occur simultaneously. Always practice in a smooth, unhurried manner, trying to avoid jerkiness. Be aware that you are working to establish more harmonious functioning of your body and mind.

When you first begin to be aware of your stiffness or lack of strength or balance, you may panic and become even more tense. You may want to struggle your way past the stiffness and fidget your way to balancing. Or else feel it's "too late" for you anyway.

Your *attitude* is the key to the successful practice of yoga. Begin realistically. Whatever you are able to do, learn to do as well as you can. Explore the quality of awareness with which you approach your "edge" (your limit, your current capacities). Learn to approach each asana with a real and healthy love for youself, with genuine gentleness and appreciation for the body that has been your faithful servant for so long.

Become aware of any tension you are carrying within you that inhibits your range of movement. With conscientious, regular practice you will gain confidence and come to explore your limitations and capacities with a playful, nongoal-oriented attitude. As you become more and more in touch with how your breathing can help you to move, you will steadily ease your way past current limitations. Flexibility will come little by little in recognizing your tightness without resisting or fighting it.

As your body loses some of its rigidity, you will discover your mind loosening up, perhaps letting go of some of its habitually limiting patterns of thought. The more relaxed and open your body feels, the more changes you will observe in your mind.

To repeat: Never tug, strain, or pull strenuously. You cannot *force* your muscles to attain desired flexibility. In performing each posture, stretch gently to where you "feel it," then hold for the number of counts recommended or comfortable for you. Should you feel discomfort in any part of your body, imagine the breath being exhaled through that area, releasing the tightness and easing the stiffness. With practice you will learn what it means to relax within the pose. If you underextend, you do not stretch the muscles; if you overextend, you damage them.

Pain

What should you do if you experience something more than discomfort and "pleasant agony"? What if the body sends out an unmistakable message of pain? In general, stop. Start again with all your attention, very slowly, with infinite gentleness. Check your breathing. Keep your body as relaxed as possible. If it begins to hurt again, stop, continuing to stretch only to the point where it hurts. (In some cases it is not advisable to stretch to the point where it begins to hurt, but to postpone that particular posture until later.) To immobilize an area of pain totally will generally result in more stiffness and pain.

Uncomfortable though it may be, there is a lot to learn from pain. *Do not ignore pain.* Like a child crying for attention, the more you ignore pain, the more insistent it becomes. But give a child your complete, undivided attention for just a few minutes and often it will run off and play. Similarly, give pain felt during an asana your total attention.

Thus, in general, stretch to the point of pain. Those asanas that especially work the area of pain should be done with extra care, but not avoided. Simple, slow movements, coordinating the movement with the breath, are generally helpful. Use your common sense or seek professional advice when severe aches or pains persist. Never take a chance on possibly aggravating any serious symptoms. (Read carefully section at beginning of Chapter 12 on "Precautions.")

Rest

Always rest in the pose of deep relaxation five minutes for every half-hour of yoga asana practice. Do not skip the pose of deep relaxation described in the asana section. Keep in mind that the body is incredibly complex, with many systems interacting to produce a given response. Relaxation after the asana practice allows the circulatory, lymphatic, respiratory, digestive, and nervous systems to make any necessary compensations to the increased stimulus from muscular and respiratory activity. (See Chapters 9 and 13 on relaxation.)

Time

The best time to practice is the time that is *consistently* best for you. In the beginning, practice at the same time each day so that your mind and body will come to expect and accept that this is what you are going to do. Choose a time with a minimum of foreseeable disturbances.

Morning practice generally gives a great feeling of having started the day out right. The mind feels more alert, and the increased circulation aids in normal, everyday functioning. In the morning the body is initially stiffer, but this does not detract from the benefits gained from the practice. Evening practice helps remove the stress of one's daily activities, and in the evening you may want to focus more on relaxation, in preparation for a good night's sleep.

It is wise to wait three hours after a heavy meal, especially if working on the inverted poses such as the Shoulder Stand. If your meals are sensible and moderate, you can begin the warm-up and stretches about an hour-and-a-half after eating, ending your practice with the inverted poses.

Whatever time you choose, set your goals realistically. Fifteen minutes a day is more beneficial than procrastinating from day to day with the idea you'll practice two hours on Saturday.

Place

You do not need a lot of space. The surroundings

should be as pleasant as possible and free of potential disturbances. Also, give yourself plenty of room; move anything you may accidentally bump into out of the way. The floor should be even. If you use an exercise mat, it should be fairly firm. Cloth-covered pads are preferable to plastic pads. The room should be around 70°—too cold a temperature may make you stiff; too hot may make you drowsy.

If you have a secluded, level place outdoors, that is ideal. Being surrounded by nature, birds singing, the soothing green color of plants, the fragrance of flowers, the warm sun—all this helps to bring your consciousness into the present and encourages attentiveness during the practice of the asanas.

The standing postures are best done on a nonslippery bare floor, with a wall to help stabilize the pose.

Clothes

The less worn during the practice of yoga asanas the better. It can be helpful to wear clothing that conforms to the shape and contour of your body without restricting movement. Some people feel most comfortable in loose cotton clothing, even though this may restrict visual awareness of the body. You can buy or make a pair of "yoga pants," which are very soft cotton pants with nonrestricting elastic or drawstring waist. Belts, buckles, and tight-waisted clothing are restrictive. Sweat pants are fine. Collars and zippers in the back of the neck can be uncomfortable.

Synthetic fibers do not allow the skin to breathe as much as cotton does, but tights and leotards have advantages. Many women (some who initially thought they were too old to wear a leotard) say just putting on their leotard puts them in the mood for the exercise aspects of yoga. Leotards now come in so many styles and colors that you are almost sure to find one that suits your taste. If at first you feel self-conscious, wear a loose-fitting cotton blouse over the leotard top.

Free Your Feet

Many yoga books, unfortunately, show the demonstrators wearing ballet slippers or tights with the feet intact. I cannot overemphasize the importance of practicing with bare feet and being able to spread your toes freely. If your feet feel cold at the beginning of a session, wear loose cotton socks that you can easily toss off. Either buy tights without feet or cut the seam (just snip the seam at the toes and roll the foot part up to the ankles). Far better to "ruin" a pair of tights than to continue ruining your feet. Take time during the day to spread your toes, and spread them often during the practice session. (Best to make it a rule *always* to wear shoes wide enought to permit you to spread your toes easily.)

Some Suggestions For "Getting in the Mood"

There are going to be days when you come up with a hundred excuses for skipping your yoga session. Legitimate reasons do happen, and all is not lost if you skip a day or two. On days when it's simply a matter of "not being in the mood," here are a few tips that may help:

A warm shower or bath before practicing the asanas is conducive to feeling more relaxed. Only be sure you don't stay in the bath to the point of drowsiness!

Sit quietly on the floor or in a chair, spine as erect as possible, and do nothing for a few minutes. You may want to remind yourself that what you are doing is one of the best things you can do for yourself and for others. Those you care about will benefit if you stay as well as possible.

If it is pleasant and quiet outside, step out before you practice or sit by an open window. Sometimes just looking at the sky helps to release our preoccupations or worries. Take time to experience the present.

You may like to hang an inspiring verse on the wall by your practice area or read a devotional poem. Some days it feels "right" to play some soothing music in the background while you practice the asanas.

Sitting or lying down, begin to listen to your breathing. Place one hand on your abdomen and one over your heart, and feel the movement of your breath flowing in and out. Be aware of your heart beating. Then consciously begin to lengthen the exhalation; the inhalation will automatically deepen as you do so. Allow this awareness of your breathing to calm and relax you. Chant "Ohm" if you like.

If your mind is full of distracting thoughts, sometimes taking a few minutes to write them down helps. If it's something you'd as soon forget, crumple up the paper and throw it away. If it's something you're afraid you'll forget, put it safely aside, then continue with your practice. If you are lucky enough to have a friend who knows how to listen, call him or her. (This is one of the big advantages of doing yoga with a friend. You can help get each other in the mood.)

Keep a yoga notebook. In it write down the asanas you plan to do, and after your practice write down what you experience, noting any changes from the day before or other observations. On the days when you absolutely don't want to practice, pick up your notebook and at least write down "nothing." This way three days won't slip by unnoticed. This is especially essential if you don't have outside yoga "connections," such as a weekly class, friends doing yoga, or yoga on TV. Your notebook and books on yoga all serve to connect you to yoga until your at-home routine is as firmly established as eating lunch.

Make a list of the most important warm-ups and asanas you want to do. Then set a timer for fifteen minutes and tell yourself you are going to do them for at least fifteen minutes, even if you feel awful inside. In that fifteen minutes the exercises and breathing may well release enough tension so that you will *want* to continue. Do a forward bend; the increased blood supply to the head may help alleviate depression.

Practice the deep relaxation described in the asana section. Then take a catnap. We have all experienced how different the world looks after renewing our energy. Remember that the practice of consciously relaxing each part of your body is legitimate "yoga," so if you do only this some days, at least you haven't missed an *entire* practice session.

12

Yoga Asanas

The yoga asanas in this section are listed in a logical sequence, and additional sequence suggestions accompany each asana description. Keep in mind, however, that the sequence given is only a suggestion and that after you become familiar with how to do each asana, you can do them in almost any order, provided you do them correctly. (Read and reread the directions.) You can discover for yourself which warm-ups and asanas are most beneficial for you.

There are many ways to vary your at-home routine. Perhaps one day do all standing poses, the next day all sitting poses, and another day all on-the-back poses. Or choose two from each category. Or one day do all of them in the sequence given.

Make it a part of your daily life to do single poses at odd moments during the day—a standing stretch before lunch, some forward bends while watching TV (during commercials), some poses on the back plus a Shoulder Stand before going to sleep.

Use common sense. The more difficult poses come easier after a few warm-ups. Remember never to force your body and to move with total attention to the response your body gives to the pose. Better to discipline yourself and do four poses consistently, every day, than to do ten poses sloppily on the weekend. The body responds positively to regularity. Fifteen to thirty minutes each day is generally better than an hour now and then. An hour a day is ideal.

Precautions

If any of the conditions listed below apply to you, we recommend that you learn the asanas on an individual basis or in a small group and inform the instructor of your condition. After you learn your body's capabilities you can join a larger group if you desire.

—Hospitalized (or had surgery) within the last year
—Injury to spine or nervous system (regardless of date)
—Heart malfunction (regardless of date)
—High or low blood pressure
—Persistent backache
—Asthma or shortness of breath
—Slipped disc (herniation)
—Sharp pain in the lower extremities
—Any other recurring disease or injury that requires a physician's attention

Whenever there is any doubt about your physical condition, it is advisable to have a complete physical examination before embarking on the practice of yoga. Be sure to tell your yoga instructor immediately if you are injured in any way during yoga practice either at home or during class. Remember that no undue strain should be felt in the facial muscles, ears, or eyes, or in breathing, during the practice. Persons with a history of heart trouble, hypertension, cerebral vascular accidents, or other serious ailments should consult their physician before attempting the more advanced inverted poses. If you feel dizzy at any time, gently bring yourself out of the pose.

After an illness resume the exercises gradually, beginning with deep breathing, the Bridge Posture, Knees to Chest, and a few gentle stretches. Add a few other postures each day.

Vulnerable Areas

Be especially attentive to the three most vulnerable areas of the body: the neck, the knees, and the lower back. When I first began yoga, I hurt my neck attempting the Headstand prematurely, I hurt my knees forcing them into the lotus, and I hurt my lower back doing too many strenuous leg lifts. An attentive, unambitious approach cannot be overemphasized.

Neck

Extreme degrees of neck flexion, extension, and rotation are not recommended. If you are in doubt as to how the neck should feel or be held during a pose, just let it be relaxed, in line with the rest of the spine. Some people can put stress on the neck area and apparently not hurt themselves, others damage their necks severely. Be very cautious if you should do neck rolls, and be very careful not to compress the neck doing postures such as the Shoulder Stand.

Remember that teachers are not perfect; they are human. Some are well trained, others are not. A teacher is there to assist you in learning the technique of the postures and to help you get the most possible benefits from your practice. But it is you who are living inside your body; ultimately you have to tune in and find out which asanas are most suitable for you.

Knees

Knees are very vulnerable. The knee joint is often sub-ject to trauma because it is a major weight-bearing joint, yet it has relatively little muscle mass around it to give it the stability of the hip, for example. For this reason it is important during your practice to keep the muscles around the knee firm. This is especially true when doing those standing asanas that additionally stretch the back of the knee. Be careful that the quadriceps muscle (anterior thigh muscle) is firm and is lending its support to the joint. Always remember to be careful with your knees. Do not force or strain them.

WARM-UPS (to be done in sequence given)

Apple-Picking Stretch:

With the feet flat on the floor (or ground), bring the arms up over the head, look up, then stretch up through every part of the body as though trying to pick apples just out of reach. Now rise up on your toes and continue reach-ing higher and higher. Relax the arms, let them fall to your sides, pause a moment, and repeat 3 times.

Rag-Doll Bend:

On an inhalation, raise your arms above your head. As you exhale, slump over from the hips very slowly, like a rag doll, bending in a relaxed manner, dangling your arms toward the floor. (Move slowly to avoid dizziness. If bend-ing should make you dizzy, skip the forward bending movements for the time being. Give your body time to be-come accustomed to new positions.) While you are dan-gling over like a loose, limp rag doll, practice breathing slowly, evenly. On an exhalation experiment with allowing your breath to help you bring your head and hands a little closer toward the floor. Then, keeping your head completely loose and your chin tucked close to your chest, come up, remembering always to move slowly. Pause for several complete breaths. Repeat 3 to 4 times.

These two exercises are excellent done first thing in the morning just after getting out of bed, or at any time during the day when you feel stiff and cramped from sitting too long.

Spinal Stretch (Plate 1):

Stand with your arms relaxed at your sides, palms turned outward. On an inhalation slowly raise your arms high over your head, interlock your fingers, and turn the palms up toward the ceiling. Try to keep your arms in back of your ears as you stretch your palms toward the ceiling. Feel yourself growing taller and taller. Take several complete breaths as you hold this position and lower your arms slowly on an exhalation. Repeat.

Side to Side Stretch (Plate 2):

Turn your palms outward, and again on an inhalation raise your arms, interlock your fingers, and turn the palms up toward the ceiling just as in the Spinal Stretch. While exhaling bend to one side as far as possible (keeping feet firm on the floor), and on an inhalation move back to the center, exhale slowly down to the other side, inhale back to the center, and slowly lower the arms on an exhalation. (Again try to keep the arms back behind the ears throughout these movements.) Repeat.

Instant Energizer (Plate 3):

(a) Stand straight with feet a hip-width apart, knees firm. Clasp your hands behind you.

(b) Inhale and move the shoulders back, lifting the clasped hands and arms as you squeeze the shoulder blades together. (Do not be discouraged if at first the shoulders are tight and the arms don't come up very far. With practice the shoulders will loosen up.)

(c) Exhale and bend forward (keeping the knees firm), bringing your clasped hands and arms up away from the back as high as they will go without strain on the shoulders. Relax the head and neck as you hold the position for several complete breaths, or 10 to 20 counts. Keep the hands clasped, arms extended, as you slowly come up on an inhalation. Relax. Repeat.

This is a favorite exercise of many people, another good one to do first thing in the morning and during the day whenever you feel like a little break. It is a very invigorating movement, stimulating circulation to the head and heart, loosening tense muscles of the back and shoulders, and stretching the legs. (Said to make a dull, lethargic person active!)

Checkpoints: Keep the legs straight, knees firm.

Wet-Dog Dance:

This is exactly what it says. Pretend you are a wet dog and shake yourself dry all over. Shake the tension and tightness out of your body. Lift and shake your legs and feet. Shake out your hands, wrists, elbows, and shoulders, letting them flop loosely as if they had no bones in them. Stand quietly with the arms loose at your sides and experience the way you feel.

Rocking:

(a) Sit up and bend your knees toward the chest, hands under the knees, curling up into a ball.

(b) Push with your feet to get some momentum to rock

back and forth on your back as you let your body go with the swing. Practice about 5 times.

(c) Hold the position where you are on your shoulders, with knees on your forehead, supporting your back with your hands.

(d) Then see if you can bring the legs and feet back behind you.

(e) When this is comfortable in slow motion, begin practicing the full rock and roll, keeping the hands in back of the knees.

Suggestions: Many people, especially those who are overweight, initially have trouble getting their buttocks off the floor. Do not be discouraged. In my classes I have never seen a person who really tries fail to get the hang of this rocking exercise and learn to really enjoy it. If you have trouble getting up and down, try this method: Lie on your back, bend and raise your knees, clasping them to your chest with both hands interlocked behind the knees. Raise your head toward your knees and slowly rock back and forth on your curved spine. With steady, patient, persistent practice you will gradually increase the length of your movements back and forth until you are able to sit with the knees clasped to your chest, feet flat on the floor, and rock back until your toes touch the floor behind your head.

Benefits: Massages and stretches the back, relieves tension in head and neck, strengthens the whole body, and increases energy.

Back Lengthening (Plate 4):

This simple exercise feels wonderful and is a preparation for the Downward Facing Dog. Great for the back and stretches the legs. Do it whenever you see a blank wall, or better yet, put your hands on a window sill or on the edge of a sturdy chair.

(a) Stand 3 to 5 feet away from the wall, feet shoulder width or more apart. Place palms on the wall, a little wider apart than the shoulders, as illustrated in Plate 4. (b) Keeping the palms firmly on the wall, try to move your buttocks as far away from the wall as possible in order to extend and elongate the spine. Work at flattening your lower back. Deepen the inhalation and exhalation as you hold the pose for several breaths.

ASANAS

Downward Facing Dog (Plate 5)— *Adho Mukha Svanasana* (*Adho Mukha*=face down; *Svana*=dog)
Sequence: Practice this *after* you get the feel for the Back Lengthening exercise. This pose is a warm-up for the other standing poses and is an excellent preparation for the more advanced inverted poses, such as the Headstand.
Benefits: This pose is especially beneficial to people who jog, run, or hike. It stretches and strengthens the legs, wrists, arms, back, increases shoulder mobility, and opens the upper back.
(Practice on a nonslippery floor or with the hands at a wall, with the inside of the thumb and index finger pressing the wall.)
(a) Come into the pose from a standing position bending the knees to place the palms on the floor. Feet and hands will be about 3 to 4 feet apart depending on your limb length and height.
(b) Position your hands wider than your shoulders until the chest can be opened freely. (You will get a feel for what this means as you practice the pose.) Feet are a comfortable distance apart, in line with the hands.
(c) As in the Back Lengthening exercise move the buttocks as far away from the head as possible—but this time

try to push the buttocks up toward the ceiling and back in order to lengthen and flatten the back. Relax the head and neck, keep the arms straight (don't bend your elbows!), and try to lower the head and chest toward the floor. (As you do this, an inverted V is formed by the shape of the body.)

(d) Work to drive the heels toward the floor. In the beginning the heels *may be way off the ground,* and you will feel an intense stretch in back of the legs. If the wrists are weak, you may be able to hold this pose for only one complete breath. Do not hold to the point that you collapse, but rather lengthen the number of breaths taken in the pose gradually until you can hold it for one minute.

Repeat 2 or 3 times. Rest in the Child's Pose, which follows.

Note: Pay attention to alignment of the hands and feet. Check that the distance between both hands and both feet is equal.

Contraindication: Sciatica

Child's Pose (Plate 6):

The Child's Pose (also known as "The Closed Leaf") relaxes the spine, eases lower back problems, and increases circulation to the face and head. It is recommended after vigorous stretching poses, to rest between poses, or for several minutes of relaxation at the end of your yoga session.

(a) Kneel on floor and sit back on heels.

(b) Rest the head on the floor in front of you. If it is not comfortable to place your head on the floor, try cradling your head in your hands, make fists with the hands and place head on top, or place a small cushion under the head. (Be sure to remove your glasses beforehand.)

(c) If not using the hands to support the head, bring them

both in back toward the toes and rest them on the floor, keeping the elbows relaxed as in Plate 6. Inhale and exhale in a natural, rhythmical way. The entire body begins to feel relaxed and restful.

Note: If the legs are tight, place a cushion under the hips, or you may find it more comfortable to place the knees a hip-width apart. Make yourself as comfortable as possible in this pose. Check that the heels are out at the side and the buttocks rest on the feet or a cushion.

Hare Pose:

Although the whole body is not inverted in this pose, in a mild way it produces the same benefits as the Headstand, increasing circulation to the head, and has the other benefits of the Child's Pose.

(a) Start by taking the Child's Pose. Lean forward until the crown of the head is resting on the floor, with the back and buttocks raised. Hands are holding the ankles. Hold as long as comfortable, inhale and exhale calmly.

(b) Do not sit straight up when coming out, but move back into the Child's Pose. Sitting back on the heels, come up slowly, back rounded, chin tucked to the chest.

Mountain Pose (Plate 7)—*Tadasana* (*Tada*=a mountain):

The Mountain Pose implies a pose in which you are standing stable, firm, still, and steady as a mountain.

Begin by learning all you can about the way you stand. Do not accept the myth that as you grow older your posture simultaneously grows worse. In as detached a manner as possible, observe yourself as you wait in line at the post office, bus stop, or store. Feel your feet inside your shoes. Is there plenty of room to spread your toes? Remember that your toes should have the same freedom as your fingers. Would you deliberately wear tight coverings on your hands that prevent you from spreading your fingers? Squeezed toes mean poor balance.

Try to tune in to the way you distribute your weight on your feet and legs. Find out if you stand with the body weight thrown mainly on one leg or if one heel is turned completely sideways. Feel if you bear all your weight on the heels or on the inner or outer edges of the feet. (Check an old pair of shoes and see where the soles and heels are worn out.)

If the weight is not distributed evenly on the feet, the rest of the body has to compensate. When the body weight is thrown mainly on the heels, you feel gravity changing; the hips become loose, the abdomen protrudes, the body hangs back, and the spine feels the strain. Then you tire sooner, and the mind does not function as clearly.

On most people—over and under fifty—postural deviations are apparent. The ideal posture is one in which both halves of the body are equal; the body looks and feels in a state of balance. It does not mean that you must strain to stand at stiff attention, exaggerating the spine's natural curve. You are working to align your spine so that a vertical line can be run from the earlobe through the shoulder, hipbone, and anklebone. If your current posture is far from this ideal, you will not be able to master the Mountain in a few days. But steady practice of the Mountain will improve your posture, and it will grow better as the days go by. Give yourself the opportunity to find out how much straighter you can stand, and do not worry about mastering all the details of the pose at once.

Procedure:
(a) Stand on a firm, even surface (on floor, not on mat or blanket). Begin the alignment process by focusing on the feet. If possible, bring the feet together, from heels to toes.

(If you have trouble balancing with the feet close together, separate them slightly.) Stretch the toes as wide as you can, open and extend them, then place them back on the floor. (If they will not spread, reach down and spread them with your fingers. Pick up the big toes and place them together.)

(b) Still focusing on the feet, close your eyes and concentrate on the way you distribute your weight on your feet. (Keep your eyes open in the beginning if you have trouble standing still with eyes closed.) Keeping the feet stationary, move the body forward slightly, back, side to side, then see if you can find the center. Try to distribute the weight evenly from the front to the back and side to side on the feet, with no weight on the toes. Again stretch and spread your toes.

(c) Next focus on the knees. Gently pull up the kneecaps by firming the quadriceps (thigh muscles). The knees should remain firm (kneecaps lifted) in all the standing asanas except when indicated otherwise.

(d) Focus on flattening any excessive curve in the lower back region by tightening the buttock muscles (as if tucking your "tail" under). (Note: Some curve is natural.)

(e) Shoulders are down and relaxed. Head and neck are in line with the rest of the spine. Your earlobes are directly above the shoulders. Feel as if someone were pulling you up by the hairs on the crown of your head. Lift the sternum (breastbone) as if to bring it under your chin.

Try to master these points one at a time without worrying about whether you will ever achieve the ideal. Daily practice will be rewarded.

Aids:

Stand against a wall.

Look at yourself in a mirror.

It helps to hang a string down the middle of the mirror.

Effects:

With steady and aware practice the Mountain becomes a relaxing, easy, and normal pose. The body begins to experience a sense of openness, free of depression and guilt. (When you are depressed, the shoulders round forward and droop. A sense of openness in the chest is related to assertiveness and humility.) With the feet firmly planted on the earth, you will feel centered, balanced, self-sufficient.

Spiritually, there is an increased sense of your connection to the earth and the heavens. The feet are well grounded, but the upper body feels light and extended upward. The earth gives support, yet you are not grasping the earth with your toes.

The Tree (Plate 8)—*Vrksasana (Vrksa*=a tree, pr. "vrik"):

Practice of balancing postures such as the Tree gives a sense of inner and outer balance, confidence and concentration. The Tree pose has a calming, steadying effect on the mind and body, and is a gentle strengthener of the legs, ankles and feet.

As you practice the pose, visualize a tree—feel the firmness of the foot you are balancing on like roots in the earth. The leg feels like a trunk, strong and straight.

Sequence: One of the first standing poses.

(a) Place one hand against a wall, raise one leg up, and place the sole of the foot against the thigh.

(b) Focus your gaze on a spot about six feet in front of you as you carefully let go of the wall and raise both arms overhead, palms together.

(c) Breathe evenly as you hold the position. Repeat and balance on the other leg.

After you become familiar with the pose practice away from the wall.

Triangle Pose (Plate 9)—*Trikonasana* (*Tri*=3, *Kona*= angle):

This pose opens the hip/pelvic area, stretches and strengthens the legs, removes stiffness in the legs and symbolizes man's connection between heaven and earth. The feet are firmly planted on the earth while the extended arm reaches for the heavens toward new ideals and destinations.

Sequence: First standing pose after the balancing "Tree" pose.

(a) Stand straight with the arms and shoulders relaxed. Step 3 to 4 feet apart. (Distance between the feet should be the length of your legs to make an equilateral triangle.)

(b) Extend the arms out at shoulder level, palms facing down. Turn the right foot out to 90° and the left foot slightly in so that the heel of the right foot is in line with the arch of the left foot.

(c) Keep both legs firm (kneecaps pulled up) as you bend to the side (toward the foot out at 90°), placing the right arm on the knee (later you will be able to place the hand on the ankle) and extending the upper arm as much as possible. Note that the extended arm is in line with the lower arm—really stretch through the fingers of the extended arm.

(d) The head is turned only slightly so that you can see the thumb out of the corner of your eye. Hold at first for only two or three complete breaths, later to half a minute. Be sure to put even weight on the back foot (by pushing down on the back foot), or the front leg will complain.

(e) Come back to a standing position with the feet still apart, change the direction of the feet, and repeat on the other side. Breathe calmly, evenly throughout the pose.

Hint: After each of the standing positions it is restful to hang forward with the arms, head, neck very relaxed.

The "Hero" (Plate 10) —*Virabhadrasana:*
This pose is named after the powerful legendary hero Virabhadra. It is a heroic posture, which builds strength, stamina, endurance, and a sense of courage. It stretches and strengthens the legs, gives balance, and teaches one to move dynamically in two directions.
(a) Stand with the legs 4 to 5 feet apart. Extend the arms out from the shoulders, palms down. Turn the right foot out to 90°, the left foot slightly in just as in the Triangle Pose.
(b) Practice keeping the trunk erect as you bend the right leg. Observe in Plate 10 how the knee is in line with the ankle (a right angle) and how the body remains erect rather than leaning over the bent knee. A mirror is helpful to check your position.
(c) Warm up the knees several times by coming down slowly to a right angle with the bent leg and back up again without attempting to hold the pose. After you have repeated this procedure with both legs, and if the legs are not complaining too much, try to hold the pose for one complete breath, gazing at the outstretched front hand. Gradually extend the number of breaths taken as you build up strength and stamina.
Hints: As in the Triangle Pose, be sure to keep the back leg firm, putting weight on the back foot by pushing down with the outside of the back foot. If the back foot slips or insists on coming off the floor, try practicing with the back foot firm against a wall.

Standing Forward Bend (Plate 11):
Forward bending brings blood to the head and is very restful when tired. Forward bending makes the legs and back more flexible and gives a feeling of "letting go."
Sequence: Between other standing poses or after the standing poses.

The forward bend position illustrated by Plate 11 demonstrates how to learn the technique of bending from the hips with the spinal column extended, as opposed to bending from the waist with the vertebrae compressed.

Procedure:

Begin by standing straight, feet about a hip-width apart. The knees are held firm—bending them is cheating! As you bend you should get a feeling of the buttocks moving up toward the ceiling and back toward the wall behind you. Concentrate on extending, elongating the spine by working to flatten the back and moving the head as far away from the buttocks as possible. In other words, you want to try to move the entire back (from the pelvis to the neck) in one unit (keeping the back straight) without compressing any vertebrae.

If the back begins to round, stop the forward movement, place the hands on the legs (*arms are straight,* as in Plate 11), and maintain this position as you focus your attention on lengthening the backs of the legs, pushing the buttocks up and back, and extending the vertebral column. (Stay in this position, if possible, for 1-2 minutes of steady, even breathing.)

To come up, tuck the chin to your chest and uncurl up slowly with the back rounded. (Later practice coming up slowly with the back straight.)

To help learn when your back is rounded instead of straight, try the following: Keeping the legs straight, bend with the back rounded from the waist. Reaching back with one hand, place your fingers on your lower back, on the spinal column, and feel how the vertebrae are sticking out (they feel like bumps along the spine). As you straighten the back, keep the fingers on the bumps of your lower back and notice how they move in as the back straightens. In forward bending the aim is not just to see how far down you can bend, but to learn to bend while keeping the spine extended, the vertebrae pulled in.

Checkpoints: Keep the knees firm. Relax the neck and shoulders. Keep weight *forward* on the feet.

Big Toe (Plate 12) —*Padangusthasana (Pada* =foot, *Angustha* =big toe)

This pose is done by standing and holding the big toes as you bend. (To be done after learning to bend with the back straight, after the back and legs have become flexible enough to attempt this pose.) As you become more flexible, move the hands further down the legs. (Note in Plate 12 that the head is moving toward a spot just *beyond* the toes, not *toward* the knees.) With practice you will be able to hold your big toes between your first two fingers and your thumbs. Always continue working to *extend* the spine. Try to pull in the lower back so as to get the abdomen in contact with the upper thighs.

Exercises on the Back.

The following exercises are good for preventing and alleviating back problems.

1. *Pelvic Tilt:*

Lie on your back with both knees bent and feet flat on the floor. Breathe calmly and relax. Deliberately press the small of your back against the floor and tighten the muscles of your buttocks (the seat muscles). This should cause the lower end of the pelvis to rotate forward. Hold about 5 seconds. Relax and repeat.

2. *Knee Presses:*

(a) Still lying on your back with knees bent and feet flat on floor, carefully grasp one knee with both hands and bring as close to your chest as possible. Hold and return to starting position. Alternate legs and repeat.

(b) Now grasp both knees and draw them toward your chest. Keep back and shoulders relaxed on the floor.

(Knee presses help align the spine and help to relieve gas, indigestion, and constipation.)

3. *Safe Leg Lifts:*

Lie again on your back, knees bent, feet flat on the floor. Breathe calmly, relax. Arms are relaxed at your side. Again draw one knee toward your chest and then straighten the leg toward the ceiling. (With practice the stiffness will leave and you will be able to bring the leg straight up to 90°.) Stretch through the heel of the foot and flex the foot (sole toward the ceiling as if standing on the foot). Hold for one or two breaths and return to starting position. Relax. Repeat several times, alternating legs.

Note: This exercise is not recommended for people with sciatic pain.

4. *Alternate Leg Lifts:*

Lie on your back with your legs straight out, knees unbent, and arms at your sides. Breathe evenly, relax. Raise one leg at a time, keeping the lower back on the floor as you lift the leg as high as you can, then lowering slowly. Repeat 5 times for each leg.

IMPORTANT LEG-RAISING PRINCIPLES:

Leg lifts, when correctly done, strengthen both the back and stomach muscles. When practicing leg lifts the point is to MINIMIZE strain on the lower back and MAXIMIZE the work of the abdominal muscles.

Keep the lower back pressed to the floor.

Bent knee leg lifts protect the back.

A Safe Way to Bring Both Legs Up.

After becoming thoroughly familiar with the preceding leg lifts you can carefully begin to lift and lower both legs.

Again lie relaxed on your back, both knees bent and feet flat on the floor. Arms are relaxed at your sides. Then bring both knees toward your chest and straighten legs toward the ceiling. Again stretch through the heels, feet flexed. To lower, bend the legs back toward chest and return to starting position. Repeat.

As you advance in your practice you can begin cautiously to practice lifting both legs straight up from the floor, holding at 90°. As you lower the legs, press the lower back to the floor. At the point where you cannot keep the lower back on the floor bend the knees or lower quickly.

In general, exhale while raising the leg, inhale or take several breaths as you hold, and exhale while lowering. Practice synchronizing the breath with the movement. Do not hold the breath.

Upright Extended Hand Foot (Plate 13):

Lie on your back with knees bent, feet flat on floor, arms relaxed at your sides. Bend both knees toward the chest, straighten the legs to the ceiling. Feet are again flexed, stretch through the heels. Lift the arms and head as high as possible. Arms are parallel to each other, palms facing each other. Keep breathing as you hold this!

Carefully lower the head and arms. Bend the knees and lower the legs. Relax and repeat.

In the beginning the legs may shake and tremble, the stomach muscles may quake and ache. With practice the pose becomes light and stable.

Bridge Pose (Plate 14)—*Sethu Bandha (Sethu* =bridge, *Sethu Bandha* =formation of a bridge)

This is another excellent exercise for relieving a tired and aching back. It also stretches and firms thighs, hips, abdomen, and relaxes the shoulder region.

(a) Lie on your back with the knees bent, feet flat on the floor, arms relaxed at your sides, palms up. Press the small of your back against the floor and tighten the muscles of the buttocks. This should cause the lower end of the pelvis to rotate forward (as in back exercise #1).

(b) Inhaling, continue to tighten the buttocks, push the soles of the feet firmly into the floor, and raise your body as high as you can. (Pushing down with the soles of the feet and pressing the shoulder blades to the floor will help you to raise up higher.)

(c) Hold for 2 or 3 complete breaths and on an exhalation slowly lower your body to the floor. When the back is on the floor, deliberately press the lower back to the floor.

(d) Pause and repeat. Check that the neck remains relaxed, lightly extended.

On-the-Back Twist—a simple form:

(a) Lie on your back, arms extended out at shoulder level, palms down.

(b) Inhale as you raise the knees up against your chest.

(c) Exhaling, lower your legs to the floor on the right (keeping the knees together) as your head simultaneously turns to the left (opposite direction). Hold for 10 to 20 counts. If one shoulder comes off the floor, press it back down. Try to keep both shoulders flat on the floor.

(d) On an inhalation raise the bent legs back up to the chest, exhale, and lower on the left as the head turns simultaneously to the right.

Repeat 3 times on each side.

(e) With the knees as close to the chest as possible, wrap your arms around the bent legs and hug them to your chest. If you can, carefully raise your head and bring your nose to your knees. Then lower the head, bring arms back to your side, and release the legs back to the floor.

On-the-Back Twist—a variation (Plate 15):

(a) Lie relaxed on your back, arms extended in line with the shoulders, palms up so that the body forms a cross.

(b) Place the sole of the right foot on top of the left knee-cap so that the arch of the foot fits on the kneecap. (The inside of the foot is parallel to the left leg.)

(c) On an exhalation rotate the entire body to the left and simultaneously move the head to the right.

(d) Hold this position for several complete breaths. Try to keep both shoulders pressed to the floor as you hold.

(e) On an inhalation move slowly back to the original position, change the feet so that now the left foot rests on top of the right knee cap, and reverse the twist to the right.

Note: Almost everyone feels confused as to which way to turn. It helps to remember that you always twist toward the side of the extended leg and the head simultaneously turns in the opposite direction.

This exercise is highly recommended following the Shoulder Stand and any time to help align and relax the back.

The Stick Pose(Plate 16)—*Dandasana (Danda* =stick or rod):

Just as the Mountain Pose is the basis from which all standing poses originate, so the Stick is the basis for all sitting poses.

The Stick Pose strengthens the legs, stretches the hamstrings, gives further awareness of the importance of an extended spinal column, straightens and strengthens the back.

(a) Sit on the floor with the legs extended straight out in front. If you have trouble keeping the back erect in this position, then sit against the wall to get a feel for extension (straightness) of the back. Or you may find it helpful to sit on the edge of a pad to help rotate the pelvic area forward and keep the back straight.Concentrate on growing "taller." (Place your fingers on the lower back to check whether or not the back is rounded. Check that no vertebrae are sticking out, just as you learned to check for straightness in the Standing Forward Bends.)

(b) Place the palms flat on the floor by your hips, fingers pointing toward the feet, to help give a lift to the back.

(c) Try to keep the legs together, press the backs of the knees to the floor. (Do not allow the knees to roll to the side, but keep the kneecaps facing the ceiling.) Note that the feet are flexed as though standing on them. As you press the backs of the knees to the floor, the heels come off the floor. Stretch through the heels.

Try to hold for one or several even breaths, pause, try again according to your capacity. With practice it will become more comfortable to sit like this.

Hints: The spine is held straight, but not rigid. (There *is* a difference.) Visualize your head like a sunflower, your back like a stem. If the knees tremble as you press them to the floor, place a small book under the heels.

Basic Full Forward Bend (Plate 17)—*Paschimottanasana (Paschima* means literally the West. It implies the back of the whole body from the head to the heels. *Tan* means to stretch, extend, lengthen out.):

In this asana you will find that the back of the whole body is intensely stretched.

Sequence: After all sitting postures. First learn the Stick Pose and the Head to Knee Pose. The procedure is similar to the Standing Forward Bends and the Head to Knee Pose.

(a) Begin the Stick Pose, then, maintaining the extension of the spine, come slowly down the legs with your hands.

Reach only as far as you reasonably can, all the while focusing on elongating the back, not worrying about bringing the head to the knees. At first, as in the Head to Knee Pose, you may first just hold your legs above the knees and work to straighten and extend the vertebral column from this position. Remember to find the *edge* of *your* stretch.

(b) When you are able to get down as far as the ankles, you can extend the spine even more by wrapping the hands securely around the balls of the feet, widening the elbows and pressing the backs of the knees into the floor.

Checkpoints: As in the previous forward bends, the bend is from the hip socket, not from the waist. Move forward over the leg as you exhale with the idea of bringing the navel toward the thigh (closing the space between the abdomen and thigh), the head toward the ankles.

Remember that one way to check if the spine is rounded is to feel it with the hand. If any vertebrae protrude, strive to extend the spine and draw them back in by raising the sternum toward the chin.

After concentrating for several breaths on straightness and extension as you move over the legs, on an exhalation surrender in a relaxing way into the pose (even if the back rounds slightly).

Come very slowly out of the pose. Pause and experience. As you learn to hold this forward bend longer, you will feel its wonderful soothing, quieting effects.

An aid is pictured on Plate 16 using a towel wrapped around the ball of the feet. Keep the arms straight as you use the "pull" of the towel to draw the shoulder blades back to expand the chest and straighten the back. As Plate 16 illustrates, you may find it easier to sit on the edge of a folded blanket or cushion for additional help in straightening the back.

When you are able to sit in the Stick Pose with the back straight, then move your hands a little way down the towel (toward the feet) and again straighten the arms, pulling back on the towel. As you progress in your practice you will be able to bend forward with the back straight without using the towel or pad (Plate 17).

After you are thoroughly "in tune" with your body's capacity, have a friend who also practices yoga hold your wrists gently and pull you forward very carefully.

Spiritually, the gesture of bringing the head to the feet represents a giving over of one's self to the divine, a gesture of humility. It is quieting, helps release anger, and holding the pose for several minutes may help relieve depression. The stretch behind the knees releases deep-seated tension. It relieves tiredness in the legs and lower back. An extended stay in this pose benefits many internal organs as well.

Head to Knee Pose(Plate 18)—*Janu Sirsasana (Janu* =knee, *Sirsa* =head):

Removes stiffness and promotes elasticity of the spine, relieves tension in the back, stretches the hamstrings, and may be beneficial to the abdominal organs. It is a quieting pose, releases anger, and teaches patience and humility.

(a) Begin in the Stick Pose. Bring the right foot to the upper left thigh so that the sole of the foot rests as close to your body as possible.

(b) Inhale and stretch arms overhead, exhale and reach down the extended leg as far as possible, holding the knee, calf, ankle, foot, depending upon the flexibility of the spine. Retain each hold 10 to 20 counts.

(c) Keeping the arms straight, the shoulder blades drawn back to expand the chest, inhale as you extend the spine (lift upward); exhale as you move downward as if to bring the head to the ankle, the more extension the better it is.

(d) Hold 10 to 20 counts, with body relaxed, surrendering to the pose.

(e) Reverse legs and repeat same process on the other side.

Note that actually moving the head toward the knees, as the name of the pose implies, is undesirable, as it may cause you to round your back. Here again, as in the Standing Forward Bends, we want to keep the back *straight,* bending from the hips, not from the waist.

Checkpoints: Exhale as you descend down the leg. Allow the breath to help you. If the back of the knee tends to come up as you extend down the leg, keep pressing it to the floor, even if you can't quite make it. The focus is on lengthening the spine. At first you may be able to bring your hands only to your thighs or knees.

As you breathe in and out while descending into the pose, it is helpful on an exhalation to visualize the tightness you feel in the back and leg softening and turning into jelly. Consciously relax and soften the facial muscles. Play with your maximum ability to lengthen and stretch.

Note: Plate 18 illustrates use of towel for the Head to Knee Pose, wrapping the towel around the ball of the extended foot. Again, keeping the arms straight, draw the shoulder blades back to expand the chest.

Contraindication: Possibly sciatica.

Bound Angle Pose(Plate 19)—*Baddha Konasana (Baddha* =caught, restrained, *Kona* =angle):

Though at the date of this writing no Western research has been done on this pose, it is recommended in yogic literature for persons suffering from urinary disorders. It may possibly enhance the health of the kidneys, the prostate, and bladder.

This pose brings relaxation and opening of the pelvis. It opens up the hips, stretches inner thigh muscles, and is a safe preparation for the classic lotus position. By practicing the Bound Angle Pose the resulting flexibility may lessen the likelihood of injury in the area of the hip joint.

Sequence: Can be done after the Stick Pose.

(a) Sit with the back against the wall in the Stick Pose. Bend the knees and bring the feet sole to sole, heels close to body. Hold the ankles or the feet. Try to retain the upward extension of the spinal column.

(b) At first the knees will probably be raised off the floor. Do not be concerned yet with pressing them down. Concentrate on sitting with the back straight. You may find it helpful to sit on the edge of a pad if you experience difficulty in keeping the vertebral column straight.

(c) When you are comfortable in this position, either with the aid of the back against the wall or sitting on a pad or without any aids, gently begin to explore your tightness as you stretch the knees and lower them to the floor. Hold 10 to 20 counts. Release the knees, pause, and repeat.

Suggestions: The mind and face should be relaxed and in a meditative mood as you hold this pose.

Placing the hands in back, as in the Stick Pose, to help lift the spine is also helpful in maintaining extension of the vertebral column in this pose. The shoulders should be relaxed, shoulder blades pulled back with the chest open. Avoid hunching over and rounding the back in a misguided effort to press the knees down.

Contraindication: Severe knee problems.

Wide Angle Pose:

This can be practiced by lying with your buttocks as close to the wall as possible, legs resting at 90° on the wall. Then carefully move your legs as wide apart as possible, keeping the entire back flat on the floor. (Be sure to move the legs apart very slowly, being careful to ease into the stretch gradually. Learn to rest in this pose for several minutes and allow the stretch to take place. The stretch is more intense when the feet are flexed. Massaging the inner thighs helps!)

Supported Shoulder Stand(Plate 20)—*Salamba Sarvangasana (Salamba*=support, *Sarva*=all, *Anga*=limb, body):

This pose is one of the greatest gifts bestowed on humanity by ancient yogis. The Shoulder Stand is the mother of the asanas. Just as a mother endeavors to bring health, harmony, and happiness to the home, so this asana endeavors to bring health, happiness, and harmony to the mind and body. It instills the virtue of a mother: patience. It also helps overcome the fear of being inverted.

If even half of the as yet unproven claims made in yogic literature are true, then the Shoulder Stand is practically a panacea for most ills of the body, considering the circulatory, respiratory, eliminative, and possible endocrine benefits.

The reverse pull of gravity eases the burden of the heart and brings a fresh blood supply to the upper torso and head. It is a marvelous posture for persons suffering from digestive ailments, asthma, thyroid disorders, and other glandular irregularities. The soothing effect on the nerves may help relieve headaches, irritability, and insomnia. It helps prevent and relieve varicosities. The change in bodily gravity may also affect the abdominal organs so that constipation is alleviated. It helps prevent constant colds, loosens up mucus in the lungs, and is also recommended for urinary disorders and uterine displacement.

Practice of this pose twice a day on a regular basis will help restore lost vitality.

Contraindications: High blood pressure. Pounding in the ears is one symptom of hypertension. For those with this condition, read step (a) carefully before proceeding.

The following steps provide the preliminary training for doing the Shoulder Stand away from the wall. They will accustom you to being comfortable and fully at ease with having your body inverted and build the strength and alignment needed to hold the pose with steadiness away from the wall. I highly recommend that you practice at the wall until you have thoroughly mastered each phase.

(a) Rest with the buttocks against the wall, elevating the legs straight up against the wall at 90°. You can scoot yourself into this position any way you like, but I suggest trying it by sitting beside the wall with the knees bent, right hip touching the wall. Pivot on your bottom so as to bring the legs up on the wall. If your bottom slips from the wall as you swing the legs up, scoot it back in.

Breathe evenly in a natural, relaxed manner. If you are unaccustomed to being inverted or have high blood pressure, I suggest you do not go on to the next step until you feel completely at ease. Those of you who are ready to move on to the next step will also benefit by remaining in step (a) 1-3 minutes or even longer. This allows the blood pressure to adjust to the inverted position.

While in position (a) check that the back of your neck is relaxed, press the shoulders down toward the floor, and release any tension in the shoulders. Consciouslessly relax each part of the face—eyes, forehead, lips, jaw, tongue, chin. Eyes may be closed; focus the attention on your breathing.

(b) When thoroughly at ease open the eyes and on an inhalation push the soles of the feet onto the wall, bending the knees, and raising the hips off the floor. Support your back firmly with the hands and bring the elbows as close together as possible.

(c) Work at straightening the back by pressing the soles of the feet more firmly against the wall. Move the hands closer to the shoulders, elbows closer together, and shift more body weight onto the elbows and shoulders.

As you straighten the body, think of bringing the chest to the chin. *Do not move your head or chin.* Do not try to bring the chin to the chest, as this movement will constrict the neck. As you gradually learn to straighten the back, the chest will naturally come to the chin.

I suggest that you do not move your feet from the wall until you can hold the pose at the wall with the back straight. Otherwise you will hold the Shoulder Stand away from the wall with a rounded back and possibly a great deal of strain on the neck .

(d) Come out of the Shoulder Stand by bringing your bottom slowly back down to the floor. It is generally beneficial to rest with the legs on the wall again for 1-5 minutes before going on to other poses. If this is the last posture you are doing, you may take part of your final relaxation this way.

Note the use of a folded blanket, placed just under the shoulders with the neck resting off the blanket. The use of a folded blanket helps to insure that there is a space between the floor and the back of the neck. This protects the neck and keeps it soft and relaxed. Thickness of the folded blanket is approximately 2 to 3 inches, depending on the angle (straightness) of your back. Width of the folded blanket should be enough to support the elbows (as illustrated).

Checkpoints: Allow the breathing to be relaxed and even while holding the pose. Experience fully how your body feels in this position. If at any time you feel in the least uncomfortable, bring the legs down immediately, but carefully. Gradually accustom your body to being inverted.

As your back begins to straighten with practice—and it

will—a straight line will be formed from chin to chest to navel to middle of the knees to the space between the feet. Keep this image in mind as you gradually work toward it.

Concentrate on keeping the back of the neck relaxed, not compressed.

Shoulder Stand away from wall (Plate 21):

(a) Lying flat on your back, exhale and slowly raise the legs 90° from the floor. Bend the knees to raise the legs when first attempting.

(b) Extend legs over head, followed by the torso.

(c) Bending arms at elbows, support the back with the palms. Think of bringing the elbows closer together while working the palms down toward the shoulders.

(d) Keep eyes open and align the big toes directly over eyes.

(e) Bring chest to chin *(not* chin to chest).

(f) Stretch through heels and hold this pose for 60 counts, increasing to 3-5 minutes or more.

(g) Bend legs at hips and lower the back slowly to the floor, vertebra by vertebra. Now lower legs to floor. (Bend the knees to lower the legs until you can keep the lower back on the floor easily.)

Checkpoints: Keep buttocks over the shoulders, head in a neutral position, back of the neck relaxed, a slight space between floor and base of neck. (Use pad under shoulders if needed.)

The Plough (Plate 22) *Halasana (Hala*=a plough):

This posture is a continuation of the Shoulder Stand and gives similar benefits. It is also an excellent energizer when you feel drained, helps relieve lower backaches. It is a withdrawing, calming pose.

Note: It is suggested that persons with high blood pressure first do the plough, then the Shoulder Stand, as this will help prevent a sudden rush of blood to the head or a sensation of fullness in the head. If in doubt, check with your doctor. *Come out of the pose if pressure or discomfort is felt.* Exercise common sense above all else.

I suggest use of the wall (best) or a chair until strength, alignment, and flexibility to do the pose away from the wall are attained.

(a) Lie on your back, head toward the wall. Adjust yourself so that the tips of your fingers barely touch the wall when the arms are fully extended behind you. (Correct distance varies; some people may need more room.)

(b) Bend the knees over the chest, then lift the legs over your head until the soles of the feet touch the wall. Position of the feet should be parallel. Support back with hands.

(c) Become accustomed to this position. If a great deal of strain is felt, bend the knees, bring them close to the face, keep legs bent as you bring them down.

(d) Extend the arms in back, interlacing the fingers. Press arms and hands toward the floor. Work toward extending and straightening the spine by lifting the buttocks up to the ceiling.

(As in the Shoulder Stand, the chin is not forced toward the chest, rather, the chest comes to the chin as the back straightens. This will prevent a sensation of choking or other difficulty in breathing so often experienced by beginners who force the chin to the chest in the Plough pose.)

(e) Hold as long as you feel at ease and are able to breathe naturally. Bend the knees, position arms beside body to help steady the force of the body coming down to floor. Keep shoulder blades back. Come down as in the Shoulder Stand, legs bent to prevent strain in lower back and alleviate tendency of head and shoulders to pop off floor.

Relax on the back or in the Knee to Chest pose.

Checkpoints: Keep knees straight. Keep feet on a height (wall or chair) if necessary to be sure the back remains straight.

Posture of Meditation (Plate 23)—*Siddhasana (Siddha* means a semi-divine being supposed to be of great purity and holiness, and to possess supernatural faculties called siddhis. *Siddha* also means an inspired sage, seer or prophet.):

The position of the crossed legs and erect back helps keep the mind attentive and alert. Siddhasana is said to be good for curing stiffness in the knees and ankles. While sitting in it the blood circulates in the lumbar region and the abdomen, which may help tone the lower region of the spine and the abdominal organs.

(a) Sit on the edge of a folded blanket with legs stretched straight out in front. Bend the left leg at the knee. Hold the left foot with the hands, place the heel near the perineum, and rest the sole of the left foot against the right thigh.

(b) Then bend the right leg at the knee and place the right foot over the left ankle, keeping the right heel against the pubic bone. With practice it will become possible to place the sole of the right foot between the thigh and calf of the left leg.

Lotus Pose—*Padmasana (Padma=*lotus):

Some of the most dedicated, finest teachers and students of yoga cannot sit comfortably in the full lotus pose. This posture is usually very hard on the knees of the average American accustomed to sitting in chairs. People in India who have been sitting this way since childhood assume the pose naturally, with ease.

The Lotus Pose is a posture for meditation and the Buddha is often depicted in it. After the knees and thighs become flexible it is a relaxing, yet alert position. The body is at rest without being sloppy. The position of the crossed legs and erect back helps keep the mind alert and attentive.

On a purely physical level the pose removes stiffness and tension in the back, knees, and ankles. (It is not good for persons with varicose veins.)

The safest preparation for the Lotus Pose is the Bound Angle Pose *(Baddha Konasana)*. *Never* yank your knees into the Lotus Pose or any other position. *(Always* treat your knees gently—learn the difference between pain and stretch.) Once injured, the knees may take a long time to heal. *Do not risk straining the knees.*

13

Savasana, the Pose of Deep Relaxation

Savasana is a genuine yoga asana and should be practiced at the end of each yoga session. It involves consciously relaxing the entire body inside and outside. As you practice it, you will discover just how quiet, calm, and relaxed your mind and body can feel. Complete relaxation brings the body to a state of homeostasis—equilibrium—which is healing to all body processes. This getting in touch with the potential stillness of the mind and body allows us to enter into a deeper state of awareness of our relationship to all life.

There are many ways to approach Savasana. I suggest that you begin with an approach most comfortable to you (which may vary from day to day) and also be open to trying new ways you may learn in a yoga class.

The Basic Procedure
  —Lie on your back on a bed or on the floor, feet slightly apart, hands at sides, palms turned upward.
  —The eyes are closed.

—Breathing is through the nose, calm, even, peaceful.

—Check your body for hidden tension in the feet, legs, stomach, hands, arms, shoulders, chest, and face.

—The lower jaw should hang loose, not clenched. The eyes should feel relaxed; the muscles of the face should be soft and passive.

—Observe your thoughts, observe that even as you lie here quietly, your mind is trying to talk to you. Allow your brain to relax, let go of all thoughts. This is *your* quiet time—all else can wait.

—Send a message of relaxation to each part of your body, from your toes to the top of your head. Take your time doing this; bring all your awareness to the part to which you send the message of relaxation. Allow your entire body to feel soft, loose, and passive.

—Lie quietly for five to twenty minutes. It is important that you come out of the pose gradually. An ideal way to come out is to roll onto one side and curl the knees toward the chest. The hands may be placed in any comfortable way, such as under the head for support or one on the shoulder and one on the knee. Remain in this position for one to three minutes, and then slowly uncurl to a sitting position. Sit quietly for a few moments, continue to experience a feeling of calmness as you slowly open your eyes.

Sending messages of relaxation: We are aware that our body responds to our thoughts. When our thoughts are tense, the body begins to feel tense. Just as when we send a message to contract the muscles, so too another message can bring relaxation to tired muscles. This relaxation message is generally known as autosuggestion or suggesting to one's own muscles and internal organs to relax. Generally, physical relaxation starts from the toes upward, and the autosuggestion passes through the entire body from the toes to the top of the head. Then, slowly, messages are sent to the kidneys, liver, heart, and other organs.

Other Suggestions for Practicing the Pose of Deep Relaxation
1. If the back is uncomfortable, place a small pillow under the knees, also a small pillow under the head or anywhere else it may help you to feel more comfortable. Cover yourself with a blanket if needed to keep warm.
2. Practice complete yogic breathing as described in Chapter 3. As you exhale, visualize all the tension flowing out of your mind and body. After several minutes allow the breathing to become more and more light and gentle; the lips may be slightly parted to get the feel of this. (Note: The arms should not be too close to the body or they may constrict the lungs.)
3. Bring awareness to how the back, the front, and the left and right sides of your body feel. The head and neck should feel aligned with the rest of the spinal column. Bring your shoulders down to the floor. Find out if you are unconsciously trying to hold yourself up. Allow your body to rest totally on the floor, to sink into the floor.
4. Become aware of your heart beat (place your palm over your heart). Be aware that allowing your mind and body to feel calm and quiet is wonderful for your heart.

Continue to allow the breathing to come freely, gently, effortlessly. Feel that your blood vessels are widening as you relax, allowing the circulation to improve without strain or effort.

Know that this is a time to allow rest and tranquillity to envelop you. Feel the warmth of your breath flowing through your entire body. Again remind yourself that there is nothing so important that it cannot wait. Let go of any distracting thoughts. This is *your time,* you should let nothing disturb you now.

5. Continue to allow your muscles to become soft, passive, *yielding;* feel them relaxing more and more as you *allow* them to do so. Let the tensions dissolve; let the body be still, at rest.

6. Surrender completely to the fact that this is your time of deep relaxation. Everything can wait. Just let the whole world, and all the thoughts that may arise in your mind, go by. Let go of all resistance to relaxation.

The Tensing and Relaxing Approach to Deep Relaxation

Tensing and relaxing all the parts of your body is a good way to get in touch with the difference in feeling between a tense and a relaxed body part. After you are familiar with the procedure and feeling of this relaxation approach, you can practice it whenever you find tension building up inside. (It can be done in a chair.)

1. Again, lie on the back with the arms and feet comfortably apart, palms facing up, feet a little apart. Close your eyes, allow all distracting thoughts to pass away.

2. Bring your attention to your feet. Feel your toes, soles, heels, and ankles. Tense your feet, tighten all the muscles, tendons, and ligaments as much as you can, then release and completely let them go. Allow them to lie motionless, to feel very loose, and then forget about them. (Note: In this and following steps, tense on an inhalation, release on an exhalation.)

3. Next, move your attention upward, going through the same tensing and relaxing process over the entire lower body: calves, thighs, hips, buttocks, and abdominal area.

4. After totally letting go of the lower part of the body, bring your awareness to your back, chest, and shoulders, and consciously allow these areas to relax.

5. Tighten your arms and hands, making fists with your hands, then lift your arms off the floor. Drop your hands and arms and let them lie soft on the floor beside you.

6. Now tighten and squeeze the muscles of your face, make a dreadful face, tighten the eyes, clamp teeth together in an exaggerated, wide smile. Wrinkle your nose. Release. Allow the mouth, tongue, jaw, to feel loose, relaxed. Gently turn the neck and head from side to side as if to say "no."

Allow yourself to discover how quiet and restful your body can feel.

14

What About the Headstand?

The Headstand—*Sirshasana:*

There are almost as many precautions concerning the Headstand as there are praises of its benefits. As with most everything else, it's not *what* you do but *how* you do it. I therefore do not recommend that anyone over fifty (or under, for that matter) attempt to learn the Headstand from directions in a book. A book has no way of judging how strong your back or neck is. And if you are able to balance upside down, the book cannot see if your body is out of alignment or if you are balancing on your forehead, which puts stress on the neck muscles. Ideally, a person of any age who would like to learn the Headstand correctly should do so on an individual basis under the watchful guidance of a knowledgeable instructor—an instructor not only knowledgeable about yoga but one who knows *you* and your capacities.

Some chiropractors have stated that the neck is not

meant to carry the full body weight, just as the shoulders are not meant to carry the whole body weight. The neck bones can deteriorate if the Headstand is practiced improperly, not to mention serious immediate injury if you try standing on your head before the strength and balance are really there. This may happen even if done against the wall. Other yoga teachers forbid it for a number of reasons, including the fact that people with high blood pressure have a tendency to burst the small capillaries in their eyes while doing the Headstand.

It must be made clear that in doing the Headstand, being able to balance upside down is not the only thing that counts. The weight is on the elbows, forearms, wrists, and hands; very little is on the crown of the head. There are as many adjustments made while upside down as in standing up straight in the Mountain Pose. The Headstand, done correctly, is actually an upside-down Mountain Pose. Learning to stand straight while right side up is an excellent preparation for learning to be straight while upside down.

I practice the Headstand daily and believe some of the benefits attributed to it are valid, recognizing that for the most part these benefits are based on the observations of yoga instructors and are not scientifically supported at the date of this writing. Some of these are: Regular practice of the Headstand increases blood flow through the brain cells, helping you to think more clearly. People suffering from loss of sleep, memory, and vitality have recovered by the regular practice of the Headstand and felt much more energetic. It can help relieve diseases of the lungs, digestive and genitourinary system. It helps prevent colds, coughs, headaches, and constipation. And it improves vision and the overall health of the body.

There are people in their seventies and eighties who still

practice the Headstand. Of course there is a difference between an older person learning it for the first time and someone who has been practicing for thirty years. Inverted poses such as the Shoulder Stand and the Hare Pose give many of the same benefits as the Headstand, as does lying on a slant board or using a Headstand device.

Under the guidance of a teacher many latecomers to yoga have learned to do the Headstand. It was reported that after the age of seventy, Israel's former prime minister, David Ben-Gurion, took up a course of yoga-like exercises, including the Headstand, to improve his physical stamina. His teacher was the noted Moshe Feldenkrais, who has written extensively on the tie-in between emotional instability and postural rigidity. After reading Feldenkrais, Ben-Gurion sent for him. In his biography on Ben-Gurion correspondent Robert St. John points out that this leader had never been interested in physical exercise. However, he was familiar with the yoga concept that man can progress intellectually and spiritually through mastery of the body.

Ben-Gurion inquired just how many lessons it would take to be able to do the Headstand and other poses. Feldenkris answered that ordinarily one lesson a week for a year would be enough, but that he had never before had a beginner over seventy.

Ben-Gurion did limber up with yogic discipline, and the results were not long in coming. For example, it was reported that he had suffered such pains in his hip joints that he awakened every fifteen minutes during the night. But soon he was able to sleep through the night. In time, he lost surplus weight and could once again do many of the things in life we take for granted until we no longer can do them—like tying shoelaces without strain. His determination undoubtedly contributed to his final mastery of the Headstand.

The Yoga Slant

The use of a slant board offers many of the benefits of the Headstand without the possibility of injury to the neck and back—or to the furniture! It is one of the easiest, most relaxing ways to stop the downward pull of gravity.

The slant position helps straighten the spine and flatten the lower back. Tense muscles become relaxed, at ease. The feet and legs, freed from their customary burden and the force of gravity, have a chance to release accumulated congestion and tension, thereby relieving swollen feet and legs. Sagging abdominal muscles get a lift, and the blood flows more freely to the face and brain. The complexion, hair, and scalp benefit from this increased circulation. Several doctors have stated that the brain functions more efficiently after the head has been lower than the feet for awhile.

Poor circulation may cause some initial discomfort. Begin slowly, adding a minute or two to your stay on the slant board each day until you can recline comfortably for ten to fifteen minutes.

You can make resting on the slant board part of your yoga routine, or lie on it whenever you feel tired during the day or before going to bed.

The cost of slant boards varies, averaging about $25.00. Many people who use them daily feel they are priceless, considering the health benefits. You can buy a portable slant board if space is limited. Or you can make one, using a board one-and-a-half feet wide and six feet long (longer if you are taller). Raise the foot end of the board to a very low chair or attach two legs to the foot end, about 12 to 15 inches high. For more comfort you can put a pad on the board.

Another way to relieve tired or swollen legs and feet is to lie flat on your back on a carpet, or on a hard, firm sofa or bed, and put your feet up against a wall, door, or piece of furniture. Put them up as high as you comfortably can. Whenever you are in a situation where you must remain on your feet for long hours, watch for an opportunity to do this exercise, if only for a few minutes. It will help prevent congestion and tension. It sounds simple. It *is* simple. But it is up to you to do it!

Instant Head "Stand"

There are several Headstand devices on the market, some more comfortable than others, and more expensive too. They can cost up to $50. I don't know of any that have been "homemade." I suggest that persons marketing these devices sell them on a trial basis, perhaps with a low rental fee to be deducted from the price of the device if the would-be headstander decides to buy it after two to three weeks.

If you have never seen a Headstand device, the only way I can describe it is as a contraption that aids a person in keeping his balance while inverted. It has a soft pad for the head and a padded support for the shoulders. It generally comes with instructions on how to use it. With a Headstand device many people are able to assume the Headstand position immediately, with the greatest of ease. But it is still necessary to accustom the body gradually to being inverted—generally, thirty seconds the first week, adding thirty seconds each week until three to five minutes a week are reached.

Persons with a history of heart trouble, hypertension, or cerebral-vascular accidents or other serious ailments should consult their physician before using the Headstand device.

Part Three

15

The Yogic Approach to Other Forms of Exercise

If one advances confidently
In the direction of his dreams
And endeavors to live the life
Which he has imagined
He will meet with a success
Unexpected in common hours.

—Henry David Thoreau

There is a connection between yoga and other forms of exercise. The practice of yoga enhances the benefits of other exercise (and other forms of exercise you enjoy enhance the benefits of yoga), whether it be running, jogging, dancing, tennis, mountain climbing, swimming, walking, or even frisbee throwing. Most forms of exercise and sport depend on coordination, balance, breath control, endurance, and a sense of physical confidence—all qualities the practice of yoga seeks to develop.

Jogging . . . Running . . . Athletics

A swimmer, surfer, skin diver, soccer player, long distance runner, and dancer named Ian Jackson explains what yoga can teach athletically inclined people of any age about physical and psychological flexibility in his exuberant book, *Yoga and the Athlete* (available from World Publications, Box 366, Mountain View, Calif. 94040, $2.50 plus .50 postage). This book relates how, after many years of ups and downs, Ian found himself on a familiar route: chronic fatigue, chronic injury, and chronic disappointment.

Just when he needed it Ian came across an article in *Runner's World.* It explained why many runners' legs hurt so much and suggested how to ease the present pain and prevent future pain by regular stretching. Its author, Joe Henderson, describes what he did.

For Joe running was a natural, smooth movement. But running had become increasingly difficult for him. He wrote: "Right now, my left heel hurts like hell. It has been hurting like that for the last seven or eight months. For several months before that, my right Achilles tendon was messed up. Before that, my right calf muscle was pulled. There have been other things."

Joe decided to look for medical help. The podiatrist quickly found out what was wrong. "Your calves are unusually strong and tight, even for a runner," he told him. "You're overdeveloped there from your years of running. Your Achilles tendon is like a rubber band that is always stretched to the point of breaking. When you put the slightest extra pull on it, something gives. Sometimes it's the Achilles itself, sometimes the calf muscle. In this case, it's the area where the tendon attaches to the heel. Unless you do something about those tight calves, you'll keep having trouble."

Joe then found out about the benefits of yoga through a running mate of his who ran the same mileage he did, but because he also practiced yoga, he didn't get injuries due to tightness.

After reading Joe's article, Ian went on to read other articles dealing with "Stretch Those Muscles." He learned that "Most active people ignore the need for flexibility. Strengthening and endurance exercises, although essential to total fitness, nonetheless act to shorten muscles and reduce flexibility. . . . Most cases of muscle tears and pulls and strains occur because of lack of flexibility. . . . Stretching by jerking, bobbing, or bouncing methods, as in calisthenics, invokes the stretch reflexes, which actually oppose the desired stretching. . . . When a muscle is jerked into extension, the natural reaction is for the muscle to jerk back, thus shortening itself again. But when the stretch is achieved slowly, as in yoga, another reaction takes place . . . which helps relax muscles being stretched."

Ian discovered he was so tight from years of running that when he tried to touch his toes, he could barely reach midway between his knees and the floor. So he immediately went out and bought himself a book on yoga and spent the first week torturing himself. His leg pains got worse. The second week he rested. The third week he reread the instructions in the yoga book, stopped struggling, and tried the *careful, aware approach.* Being relaxed and noncompetitive made all the difference. His body became loose and flexible; he began to experience a feeling of weightlessness, lightness of body, and light-footedness. In *Yoga and the Athlete* he explains just what Yoga does.

There are many similarities between running and yoga. For instance, rhythm is important to both. Once you have perfected the asanas, you can practice them in a certain combination and with a rhythm that prevents the development of fatigue. . . .

Avoiding over- and underextenstion is also important. If you underextend, you do not stretch the muscles. If you overextend, you damage them. In running, if you do too little, you do not improve. If you do too much, you damage the heart, the tissues, and the muscles.

If you practice sport as yoga, as a way of becoming aware of the body, you can develop the kind of sensitivity a skilled surgeon has. Yoga also brings deep relaxation. It can be used to stabilize your energy before competition and after.

A Yogic Approach to Walking

Walking, like breathing, is something we take for granted until we can no longer do it without effort. If you walk with awareness—that is, not ten steps ahead of yourself, thinking about what you have to do when you get home— then walking becomes a meditation.

Walking provides a natural opportunity to observe your breathing. As we've stated, far too many people are shallow breathers. While you will exhale enough oxygen to stay alive, unless you consciously deepen your breathing while sitting still, you will not be breathing deeply enough to help overcome the feeling of drowsiness in the mid-morning or mid-afternoon. As you walk, you naturally begin to deepen your breathing; if not, you become breathless.

When you walk, practice breathing slowly, evenly, inhaling and exhaling in a definite rhythm. You can approach this by controlling your breathing as you count steps. For example, inhale as you take four to six steps, exhale on the next four to six steps. This rhythm will, of course, vary from person to person, also from day to day. At first you may only inhale two, exhale two. Try to maintain the same number of steps on each inhalation and exhalation.

Like anything else new, it may feel awkward in the beginning, a waste of time when you have more important things to think about. Play with it, give it a chance. As you practice, you will find your lung capacity increasing. The length and speed of your walk will, of course, affect your rhythm of breathing. But after awhile you won't need to count, and you will naturally breathe deeply and rhythmically. Practicing such rhythmic breathing will help you walk with a more relaxed, balanced stride, which in turn will make walking more enjoyable and invigorating. Also, being conscious of the breath, breathing calmly, will enhance the mind-clearing effects of walking and bring your consciousness into the present.

If you need additional motivation, remember that the stimulation of the circulation and breathing that occurs in walking contributes immeasurably to the elimination of wastes from your body.

Approach walking just as you do the yoga asanas. Begin realistically, according to your capacity. Like your yoga practice, it must be done properly to derive the most benefits. Stand on any busy city corner and you will see there are almost as many odd ways of walking as there are personalities.

First, allow your head to follow your body. People who tend to live in the future often walk with their heads and necks sticking out. Of course, the future never materializes, and they start to feel that life is passing them by.

Just as you bring your awareness to your breathing as you walk, give attention to your spine. If you can walk, you can improve the way you walk. Be aware of how you hold your head. Which way do your feet point? Keep the chest up and open to help align the spine. Do not raise the shoulders, but keep them back and down—remember, this is not an exaggerated military posture. Allow the relaxation that should come from walking to take place. (If necessary, slow down your stride temporarily and focus on walking correctly.)

Wear loose, comfortable clothing. And be sure to wear low- or flat-heeled shoes that give sufficient support for walking on hard concrete, and wide enough to let your toes spread comfortably. Ideally, walk in a grassy area. To toughen up feet that have become tender, take a child along and follow its example when it kicks off its shoes to walk and run with more ease.

Walking, followed by a 10- to 20-minute yoga session, is an ideal combination. If you should overdo it on some of your walks, rest afterward, feet up against the wall or on a slantboard. Then, when rested, do a few of your favorite stretches.

It is tiresome at any age to stand on your feet all day. If your feet or legs start swelling from too much standing or sitting, prop them up. When standing or sitting, there isn't enough pressure in the veins of your legs to push the blood back up to the heart efficiently. Walking gets the blood circulating again.

A Word on Fast Stretches

Fast, vigorous stretching exercises are not effective in keeping your muscles flexible. All stretching exercises, whether called "yoga stretches" or something else, should be done slowly, with awareness, allowing the muscles to relax, release tension, let go. Forceful bouncing, bobbing, and frantic pulling in an attempt to stretch out tight muscles will not make you more limber. On the contrary, the muscles become tighter.

When doing stretching exercises, such as bending or

twisting at the waist or hips, trying to touch your toes, move slowly. When you have reached as far as you can, hold that position for at least a few seconds, just as you do in the yoga postures, and allow your breathing to relax you. It is valuable to repeat the exercise and hold it a little longer the second and third time.

Miscellaneous Myths and Pointers

Some people are under the impression that when certain muscles are exercised (given a workout), the fatty tissues (deposits) in that corresponding area are "burned up." For instance, the best way to trim excess inches around your middle might be to do sit-ups and leg lifts. It does seem that certain exercises are more effective for certain areas of the body, but exercise "experts" now believe that exercise burns fat from all over your body and not from one specific area, regardless of the type of exercise. This isn't so bad, as those of us who are plump around the middle would usually like to slim down in other areas as well.

Neither is it necessary to "work up a good sweat" to benefit from exercise. The purpose of perspiring is to lower the body temperature to prevent overheating. You may weigh slightly less after a sweaty workout, but this is because of water loss, which is promptly replaced when you drink a glass of water to quench your thirst.

Resistance exercises, especially when done in a yoga-like manner, such as push-ups and chin-ups, or any other activity in which the body is pitted against a hard-to-move object, increase strength in the person over fifty. If you do them sensibly and regularly, you can actually become stronger in your later years than ever in your entire life! Although the maximum potential for strength decreases somewhat as one grows older, through practice a much higher percentage of one's potential may be reached.

Whatever form of exercise you choose, you should not end up panting for breath or with your heart pounding or with a sense of fatigue. Should any of these conditions prevail and linger beyond a short rest period, you are overexerting yourself. Better to cut whatever you did in half and do the rest the next day. Exercise should be a refreshing experience.

16

Yoga, Nutrition, and Your Well-being

Better is a dinner of herbs where love is than a fatted ox
and hatred with it.
—Proverbs 15:17
Better is a dry morsel with quiet than a house full of feast-
ing with strife.
—Proverbs 17:1

Keeping It All In Perspective

Yoga and good nutrition are two powerful, natural healing tools, each lending support to the other. Yoga enhances the effects of nutrition by aiding the assimilation of
nutrients and by facilitating elimination of waste products.

And a "right-for-you" nutrition program can enhance the effects of yoga by helping to break down and clean out waste deposits that make the body stiff—and by giving energy to do the asanas!

Being involved with yoga encourages sensitivity to the dietary needs of our bodies. The awareness yoga brings helps us cast off entrenched patterns of habit, including overeating and compulsively demanding certain taste sensations. The practice of yoga, by bringing our consciousness into the present, encourages us to observe ourselves as we eat. When you do indulge in pie and ice cream, for example, rather than pretending to yourself you're not overeating again, give eating the pie and ice cream all the awareness you can muster. Let go of guilt feelings and enjoy your "indulgence" to the fullest. Make eating a celebration. Be alive to everything you are doing—smelling, tasting, chewing. Savor each mouthful with all your senses as it tastes now, not just as the memory of how it tasted in the past.

Food As a Key to Mental Health

Food is a key to mental health inasmuch as optimal nutrition increases the ability of the body to cope with influences from the outer environment. A person's internal climate is largely responsible for the way the external environment affects his physical and emotional health. In their book *Psychodietetics* (Stein and Day, New York, 1974), Dr. E. Cheraskin and Dr. W.M. Ringsdorf, Jr. say:

Medical investigators have known for many years that severe nutritional deficiencies cause severe mental illness. In recent years, a number of innovative researchers examining less serious mental conditions have found evidence that the twilight zones of emotional stress are also caused or worsened by the malfunctions of the body's nutritional machinery. Most recently, a few researchers have discovered that certain people are *genetically predisposed to extra special nutrient needs.*

. . . Sound biochemical principles underline the food-to-mood phenomenon . . . Dietary nutrients have a profound influence on the way we feel, think and respond to and perceive the world around us. . . . Nutritional therapy should be used as an adjunct to all other forms of mental therapy.

Nutritional therapy does not provide the insight and emotional understanding many people still need once their metabolic imbalances are corrected . . . Standard psychological therapy is most valuable when the patient is no longer the victim of distorted metabolic perception.

Breaking the "Fast"

Breakfast means to break a fast, and since your body has been fasting during the night (provided you did not raid the fridge at 2 A.M.,), the body is undergoing a cleansing process. A prime sign of this is waking up in the morning with your tongue and mouth coated and a general feeling of sluggishness.

It is therefore generally advisable for most people (not all) to begin each day with a liquid that enhances the body's cleansing process. The juice of a ripe lemon (preferably tree-ripened) in a glass of water or in your favorite herb tea sweetened with a little raw honey is one of the most beneficial ways to break your night's fast. The amount of vitamin C in a lemon may be minimal compared to a high potency pill, but its quality is infinitely superior.

If you use unsweetened, bottled fruit juice (apple, grape, prune), adding a squeeze of lemon will restore some of the enzyme value destroyed when the juices were heated and bottled. Dilute the juice with about half spring water. (Avoid canned juices, as they may be contaminated with lead. About 30 per cent of the dietary intake of lead reportedly comes from canned foods.)

A Cold Shower?

After a refreshing, cleansing drink, taken about a half-hour before breakfast for optimum benefit, it's time for a warm bath or shower, followed by a rinsing of cool water. Brrrr, you say? You've probably heard some of the stories about robust eighty-year-old Europeans who go rolling in the snow and swimming in half-frozen lakes every morning. And here in the U.S. we have various groups of hearty folk past sixty who thrive on winter swims in the ocean. It is advisable to ease the body gradually into a heartier state. Begin by ending your warm shower with a lukewarm shower that gets a little colder every day, and just before you get out, let cold water run over your neck and face. Cold showers do tone up the body, stimulate circulation and help build resistance against colds, but trying to shock the body back into shape is not recommended.

Breakfast: Lighter and Less Sweet

What to eat for breakfast depends a great deal on the six W's: the weather, your waist, your whim, your will, your work, and what you have in the house to eat.

Watch the way different breakfasts make you feel. Do a couple of eggs on toast wake you up and keep you going all morning? Or does this combination put you back to sleep, indicating, perhaps, that for you a lighter breakfast of fruit with yogurt, or some light soup, for example, is more suited to your organism?

I have yet to meet a person who doesn't look sleepier after a big bowl of granola. Granola is a transitional food, better than cornflakes or doughnuts and coffee, but not as substantial nutritionally as a simple, easy-to-digest whole grain cereal like millet or brown rice. Most commercial granola brands contain cooked oils plus sugar, two items to avoid if you wish to keep your arteries unplugged, and there's no telling how old the ingredients are. If you're fond of granola, make sure the ingredients are fresh—or make your own at low temperature (don't overheat the oil) and chew it well.

Much of the protein research in this country was conducted by meat and dairy interests, so naturally their products came out on top. In general, though, it is advisable to choose some form of high quality protein for breakfast. In terms of NPU—Net Protein Utilized—whole grains, seeds, and nuts are equally useful. Eaten raw, sprouted, or properly cooked (whichever is appropriate), these three foods are sources of essential unsaturated fatty acids and lecithin, both considered to be important in normalizing blood cholesterol, and are also a dependable source of vitamin E and B-complex. The bran of grains and seeds is recognized as being vital to the normal function of the digestive organs and for the prevention of such diseases as appendicitis, diverticulitis, and cancer of the colon.

Eat Less

No one said it better than Benjamin Franklin when he remarked that "a full belly is the mother of all evil."

Russian statistics show that all their centenarians are moderate eaters. Dr. C.M. McCay, of Cornell University, has demonstrated scientifically that overeating is a definite and principal cause of disease and premature aging. On the other hand, moderate eating can extend life and prevent disease. "The thin rats bury the fat rats."

Unfortunately, due to the ready availability of overrefined, easy-to-swallow-without-thinking-or-chewing foods, we tend to be overfed but undernourished. Food eaten in excess of actual needs interferes with proper digestion and assimilation. Overeating, especially when the food is not thoroughly mixed with saliva, causes fermentation, gas, and putrefaction in the intestines and inadequate assimilation of the nutrients in the food. Occasional indulgences, followed by a nap and then a walk and a yoga session, can be tolerated by most of us. But always remember that moderation will improve the assimilation of what you eat and that *it's not what you eat but what you assimilate that counts.*

Yoga and the Digestive System

It is clear from a reading of authoritative texts on yoga that the authors were keenly aware of the digestive system. For example, in one of the great books, *Hatha Yoga Pradipika* (written by Svatmarama Suri in the seventeenth century), there are continual remarks concerning effects of certain yoga practices on the "gastric fire."

Many yogic practices are claimed to have beneficial effects on the digestive tract. For instance, the practice called *agnisara* is recommended to treat dyspepsia (indigestion) due to hypoacidity. *Agnisara* is performed by exhaling completely, then gently pushing the abdomen inward and outward alternately for as long as the breath can be comfortably held out, followed by a gentle inhalation. It is believed (not proven) that this practice stimulates secretion of digestive enzymes and, presumably, secretion of hydrochloric acid in the stomach to help better digest food. *Agnisara* may also stimulate general peristalsis (propulsive movements) of the digestive tract, and is therefore recommended in helping to alleviate constipation.

During another practice, *uddiyana bandha* (better known as stomach lift) and *nauli* (alternate or simultaneous contractions of the two rectus abdominus muscles of the abdomen), the large intestines are moved around considerably. It seems likely that this would aid in mobility of fecal contents through the large intestine. (These exercises are also recommended to prevent and treat constipation and may be learned from a yoga instructor.)

Aswini mudra (rhythmic contraction of the anal sphincter muscles—the levator ani) helps tone the muscles of the abdomen and pelvic floor, and is therefore believed to prevent constipation and also hemorrhoids. It has also been reported that *aswini mudra* has cured retroversion of the uterus (provided there were no fibrous adhesions in the pelvic area). As retroversion of the uterus can cause constipation, relief of such uterine displacement by *aswini mudra* can relieve constipation.

Colon Health

Mental clarity comes from a clean colon and a straight spine.
—Old Hindu Proverb

Good colon health starts in the same place digestion starts—the mouth. Most of us know that we should chew, chew, and chew some more until our food turns to mush. But haste, habit, nerves, often make us careless.

So the first suggestion is to take time to observe your own chewing patterns. Usually, after only ten chomps or so the epiglottis at the rear of your mouth dilates automatically and allows the food to drop prematurely into the esophagus. Knowing WHY you should chew may motivate new habits.

Chewing does more than chop food into smaller pieces and mix the saliva with food, which is the beginning of the first stage of digestion and breakdown of foods into different elements and fuels. As you chew, the chemical reactions that take place in the mouth with the saliva are now believed to trigger the brain to call out the necessary action from the body required to process the food.

Chew, Chew, and Chew Some More

Without going into a long treatise on enzymes, it will suffice to say that the first enzyme, ptyalin, is found in the salivary glands. It is extremely important that all starch-containing foods, such as rice, bread, potatoes, and corn, be thoroughly masticated and mixed with the saliva in the mouth before swallowing.

Ptyalin works on starch all the way down into the small intestine. No other enzyme works on the starch until it goes beyond the stomach into the small intestine. If sufficient salivary ptyalin has not had a chance to reduce initial starch molecules to dextrin, then the pancreatic enzyme that meets it later will have to work harder to complete digestion.

This is just one more way we put undue stress on our bodies and wear them out prematurely. Neglecting to chew starches thoroughly is one of the common ways we abuse the food value of the carbohydrates and cheat ourselves of its nutrition. (Yes, chewing can lower your grocery bill like nothing else. You will eat less and assimilate more.)

There is no enzyme in the body to break down cellulose. The colon will eventually use the minute bits of cellulose broken up in chewing as a broom to sweep the waste products of digested food out through the rectum. But if cellulose, found in most vegetables and in cereals, whole wheat, bran, is not broken up thoroughly, it can have just the opposite effect in the digestive tract. Blockages may occur, causing gas, putrefaction, bloating, and other discomforts.

Salads and Colon Health

Fresh vegetable salads are ideal for building overall health, and especially colon health, but the amount should be governed by your ability to handle cellulose. YOU MUST CHEW RAW VEGETABLES THOROUGHLY. If, however, you are not a thorough chewer or have trouble chewing, or if, no matter how well you chew, you still feel you cannot "handle" digesting raw vegetables, then you would be wise to invest in a raw juice press. Though expensive, in terms of a preventive medicine investment, a juicer is priceless. Many natural food stores carry freshly made vegetable juices.

Steamed vegetables, cooked at low heat just long enough to break down the cellulose, should be included in the diet when possible.

The second suggestion for colon health is to tune in when those two faithful friends, your pancreas and liver, say they need a little time off from more meals. The liver and pancreas are the two glands whose secretions complete the breakdown of food energy into body energy.

If these two organs are weakened by congestion, they will not function properly. Knowing when it is time to fast on herb tea, diluted fruit juices, or other cleansing foods will give these two deserving guardians a chance to restore themselves so that they can serve you even better when the next meal comes along. Even skipping one meal and eating moderately the next helps a lot.

Third, work with the rhythms nature establishes in our bodies. When unhindered by disease, digestion and metabolism try to establish their specific rhythms, and elimination tries to do likewise. Eliminating waste matter at regular intervals aids and encourages the body's nutritional cycles. Eating at approximately the same time every day (not too many midnight snacks), balanced with rhythmic elimination, plays a major role in protecting the cells against destructive congestion and aids nutrition in getting to all the tissues and organs of the body.

Some Personal Thoughts On Not Eating Meat

For me, not eating meat is now as easy and natural as eating meat once used to be. About ten years ago I met some vegetarians, and their ideals felt right. It was never a struggle to "give up meat," rather *it* gave *me* up.

The decision to abstain from meat should come from an honest desire—from within you—not something forced because now you are doing yoga or whatever. Although giving up meat is not a prerequisite to beginning the practice of yoga, I would encourage you to experiment with vegetarian dinner entrées (there are more nonmeat cookbooks on the market than ever) and give the subject of eating less meat the attention it merits.

Nutrition Do's and Don'ts

DO:

1. Eat natural foods, and eat them raw or cooked at low temperatures whenever possible.
2. Drink certified raw milk where it is available. Goat's milk is really great. Cultivate a taste for easy-to-digest milk products like yogurt, buttermilk, and kefir.
3. Eat only foods that will spoil, and eat them before they do!
4. Use foods from the sea regularly—fish and also sea vegetables, which come in easy-to-use, dried form.
5. Use fertile eggs from ground-fed chickens (happy ones!) when you can get them.
6. For shortening in baked goods use unrefined soya, sesame, peanut, or safflower oil with no preservatives.
7. Use safflower oil for frying, as it has the highest smoke point of good oils.

Unrefined olive oil is excellent on salads.

8. Learn to make your own ice cream and yogurt, or buy ice cream and yogurt made from natural ingredients.
9. Drink water, milk, natural fruit juices, herb teas in place of other beverages. Make "soft drinks" out of carbonated or mineral water and unsweetened fruit juice.
10. Use carob, which is naturally sweet, for chocolate-like flavor.
11. Find a source for organically grown fruits and vegetables if at all possible. If you have space, grow your own. Grow sprouts on the kitchen counter.
12. Use only cooking utensils that enhance rather than detract from the food's potential value, such as stainless steel, enamelware, glass, or iron.

DON'T:

1. Don't eat highly processed foods such as sugar, white bread, cookies, crackers, TV dinners, or concentrated synthetic protein drinks.
2. Don't use processed milk. (pasteurized, homogenized, dried, or canned).
3. Don't eat foods containing chemical preservatives, dyes, artificial coloring.
4. Don't overuse any one meat, such as beef in steak, roast, hamburger, meat loaf, casseroles. Don't constantly use the muscle meats, which are the least nutritious part of the animal. Use organ meats instead—liver, heart, kidneys.
5. Don't use eggs produced by hens in small cages, force fattened, and sprayed with insecticides.
6. Don't use deep-fat frying, as fatty acids break down at high temperatures. Avoid doughnuts and french fries in particular, as well as other fried foods.
7. Don't use hydrogenated shortenings and heat-treated oils with preservatives. Avoid margarines.
8. Don't use commercial milk products that contain artificial coloring, flavoring, emulsifiers, or sweeteners.
9. Don't drink soft drinks with or without sugar; avoid stimulating drinks that exhaust the adrenals.
10. Don't use chocolate, as it interferes with mineral utilization and is highly allergenic.
11. Avoid (if at all possible) fruits and vegetables that have been sprayed, fumigated, dyed, or waxed. Fresh is usually better than frozen, frozen better than canned. Avoid oversweetened canned fruits.
12. Don't cook in aluminum. Be careful not to overheat teflon, and try not to scratch your pans.

17

Two New Directions for People over Fifty

About three years ago a handful of southern Connecticut residents, all older people, began to meet regularly in search of a positive approach to aging. They were aware of the fact that the second half of life can't be played the same way as the first. And hobbies and weekly bridge games at the senior citizens' center weren't enough. They formed a group called the Phenix Society. Its director is John White, author of *Frontiers of Consciousness* and editor of *The Highest State of Consciousness*. In an article in the March, 1976, issue of *East West Journal* he wrote:

> They'd all experienced midlife crisis—that time when the values and game plans of youth lose their luster, and apathy or depression can set in with a consequent loss of physical and mental vitality. So their weekly gathering centered around reading, discussion, and meditation in their quest for wisdom and serenity.

Thus the Phenix Society was born—"Phenix" because it is the immemorial symbol of renewal. And now, rising from the ashes of burnt-out lives, there are nearly a score of Phenix Clubs from coast to coast, with a total membership of several hundred, sponsored by the parent organization, the Phenix Society. Since twenty million Americans are over sixty-five and sixty million are over forty-five—most of them in the same existential bind as those Connecticut people—there is an obvious need for such an organization. But no one else seemed to offer anything of this sort until the Phenix Society began to function.

Carl Jung wrote in *Modern Man in Search of a Soul:* "A human being would certainly not grow to be seventy or eighty years old if this longevity had no meaning for the species to which he belongs . . . We cannot live the afternoon of life according to the program of life's morning."

Reading this passage was one of the key events that helped to bring the first Phenix Club to birth in Guilford. Its attending "midwife" was Jerome Ellison, then sixty-seven and nearing the end of a two-decade career in education as a professor of English.

"During the 1950's, a group of people, of whom I was one, was going through what is now known as midlife crisis," Ellison says. "At the time, the only handy name for it was 'maladjusted.' The prospect of aging seemed extremely bleak, and we faced it without joy. Since it was inevitably coming our way, however, we decided to see what we could find out about it."

The result, some twenty years later, is the Phenix Society and its local Phenix Clubs. A brochure describes the Phenix experience as "a mature adventure." The Phenix Society, it says, is "a friendship association of men and women who seek to improve the quality of their lives. The philosophical and spiritual requirements of the second half of life are its central concerns."

Each meeting begins with a short period of silence in which members generally meditate, although it's not required, (New members get meditation instruction from old ones.) Then a discussion follows, led by a different member each week. This helps to develop leadership qualities in everyone and keeps an individual member from dominating or building a cult. Discussion is usually based on a selection from the Society's handbook, "The Last Third of Life Club" (Pilgrim Press, 1973), which contains twelve "conditions of being" to guide club members in their progress to joyful, creative living. These conditions, or steps along the path of growth, are as follows:

1. We admit that death is closer for us who are in the last third of our lives than it is for the average person; that in this respect we are different from the majority of people.

2. We have come to see that, for those who are prepared, the eventual passage from this life can be a glory rather than a dread.

3. We have decided to use our remaining years primarily for this preparation.

4. We assert that the last third of life is given by nature for this high purpose; that it can illuminate earlier experience in joyous fulfillment of a rounded life.

5. We have resolved to give over our lives to Cosmic Creative Intelligence as we individually name and experience this divine force.

6. Through regular morning and evening meditations, we are finding ourselves more and more in harmony with this transcendent Power.

7. Reviewing our past in the company of other Last Thirders has shown us that our earlier life goals no longer suffice.

8. Through reading, discussion, and reflection, we have humbly attempted to discover and cultivate those higher values that are essential to our new life.

9. Having thus gained a clearer perspective on life's major phases, we have steadfastly sought the wisdom it is the business of life's later years to acquire and preserve.

10. These steps have brought an awareness of cosmic dimensions we had not hitherto explored and have led us into the realm of deep spiritual experience.

11. Though aware that the workaday world under-values spiritual wisdom, we offer what we have of it when asked.

12. As our special responsibility, and as opportunity offers, we carry to others in the final third of life the heartening word that seniority can be joyous.

No one is required to believe anything, of course. The conditions may be personally meaningful, but at the very least they serve as key topics for discussion in the search for meaning.

After the meditation period, the evening's leader makes some opening remarks for ten or fifteen minutes, sharing his or her insights, agreements or disagreements, and practical application of the passage chosen. There follows a round-table discussion that is often far-ranging, therapeutic, and profound. Not the sort of stuff you get at cocktail parties or lonely hearts clubs. It's the kind of talk that literally heals, as was the case recently with one Connecticut chapter that met each week in the home of a member with terminal cancer. Two months after meetings began in his home, he was up and about his business. The club isn't making any claims for itself, but the fact is that they taught the patient a meditation technique for healing himself, and then offered supportive friendship.

Each meeting formally lasts no more than an hour and a half, but members often linger because something beautiful is happening and they are reluctant to just drop it suddenly—not when it's vital, not when it's getting to you where you live.

Ellison, who wrote the society's handbook, is writing a new book entitled "The Best Is Yet To Be," which is a practical handbook based on Phenix Club experiences. The Society has also offered a course entitled "A Philosophy for the Middle Years," intended for college use in continuing education programs, which are usually well filled with older students. Four major universities (Virginia, Iowa, Texas, and Missouri) have adopted it.

Why the need for a new book and a college course? Although the Society originally saw the problem of quality in life as something special to older people, it soon found that practically everyone had that hunger. In no way was this need limited to "the last third of life." Middle-aged people, newlyweds, college students, the lonely, those who might otherwise be swamped by midlife crisis, pre-retirement stress, post-retirement slump— they were all looking for something that would help them become more creative and fully functioning.

It seemed natural, therefore, to extend an invitation to anyone who was interested. Now there are four Connecticut chapters of the Phenix Society. Others are operating in New York City, Jacksonville, St. Louis, Kansas City, Colorado Springs, San Diego, Phoenix, and San Francisco; and still others are forming in various parts of the country.

Each chapter operates independently in matters of finance. It costs nothing to join and there are no dues, but people are advised to buy the handbook. For information write: The Phenix Club, P.O. Box 25, Guilford, CT 06437.

Phenix Clubbers are those who are thoughtful about living and concerned about midlife crisis. When the children are out of the nest, when you've achieved material success, what do you do for an encore? That's when people find that the second half of life can't be played the same way as the first. And that's what Phenix Society people aim to do something about, by keeping their minds alive and inquiring rather than watching the pre-retirement blues set in as they reach for the bottle and contemplate suicide.

To help people stay alive and vital, Phenix Clubs have also sponsored public lectures, weekend retreats, meditation instruction, and a pre-retirement seminar for business executives.

In addition, there is an ongoing Wisdom College, a very inexpensive four-year correspondence course in which anyone can enroll at any time. It uses inexpensive books (one per month) to form a curriculum based on "the greatest insights won by ten thousand years of civilization largely ignored by existing schools and colleges." The faculty of four are professors at Connecticut colleges and universities.

"We older people have been conned out of our real function in life by the youth cult," says Ellison. "Youth isn't the only hope of the world. Humanity's hope lies in the wisdom of age. Clearly, then, we must revise the national attitude toward aging. The notion that a person is through at thirty, fifty, or sixty-five or any age is just plain nonsense. Nature wouldn't have given us extra years past the productive phase of child-rearing and householding if they didn't have meaning. The Phenix Society attempts to explore that meaning. And it helps amazingly to realize that one does not have to go it alone, or be puzzled about the path."

> Grow old along with me!
> The best is yet to be,
> The last of life for which the first
> was made.
> —Robert Browning

Another outstanding example of the change that is happening all over America is the SAGE (Senior Actualization and Growth Exploration) project. Judging from the project's overwhelming success, SAGE's message is one that people have been waiting to hear for quite some time. An article by Laughingbird in a recent (#9) issue of *New Age Journal* describes what it is and what it is doing.

In January of 1974, Gay Luce, a Berkeiey, California, psychotherapist, well known for books *Sleep* (Pyramid, 1972) and *Body Time* (Pantheon, 1971), piloted a project designed to revitalize the elder years, using a variety of yoga, meditation, and body awareness techniques. Gay was inspired to start SAGE after taking an intensive human development training program at Nyingma Institute. The program, which used Tibetan Buddhist meditation, relaxation and awareness techniques, was given to a group of medical, psychological, and therapeutic professionals by Lama Tarthang Tulku. Gay was especially interested in Lama Tulku's description of attitudes toward old age among Tibetans, who regard it as the richest time for inner growth and contemplation—a time for looking over life experiences, sharing them with younger people, and preparing for a good death. Gay wondered if the awareness techniques could be used to counteract our own culture's terrible neglect and devaluation of the experience of old age.

She began exploring a positive approach to aging with a 74-year-old friend, Helen Ansley. Helen reacted so favorably to the yoga, breathing, and massage exercises they practiced together that Gay was encouraged to start the first SAGE group—a dozen people aged 65 to 95.

SAGE uses a wide range of techniques to help shake off negativity toward old age and to encourage positive action. Among its tools are art therapy, autogenic training, biofeedback, Feldenkrais exercises, foot massage, Gestalt dream analysis, guided imagery, Hatha Yoga, meditation, music therapy, visualization, breathing therapy, and Tai Chi.

Worden MacDonald, one of the original members of the SAGE group, explained what Gay was trying to do in those early days of SAGE. "When we first started, Gay was exposing us to some of the things the 'young people' are into. Deep breathing was a big part of it. We did a little Tai Chi and a little yoga. I think she just wanted to see if old people could respond to new things as young people do. Most of us have changed considerably for the better. It's a good thing: it makes us feel good . . . *Our society is very adept at making people miserable and unhappy . . . The whole idea of SAGE is to refuse to be old, scared, pushed around or told you're too old or can't do anything.*"

Mac was trying to get used to his new hip replacement when he first came to SAGE meetings. "It was a pretty scary thing to realize that my leg wasn't my leg at all, that almost down to my knees was a piece of plastic and it was fastened onto my pelvis, and I thought they put the whole thing together with Elmer's glue, and it would probably come apart. So every time I heard an extra squeak, I thought 'Oh no, this is it, it's coming apart.' . . . I was still using a cane when I started to come to SAGE, and they started me on balancing exercises. It's remarkable what happens with complete relaxation. I'm gettin' so I can stand on one leg pretty good and wave the other one around."

Another woman, Eleanor Karbach, 73, described herself as an "old post-cancer case with high blood pressure." She had a great story about how she stopped a case of tachycardia (rapid heartbeat) with yoga. "I had been to a party, eaten the wrong things, and went to bed when the attack came. I did yoga breathing and the attack passed. It was a miracle." Ellie learned at SAGE how to warm her entire back in twenty minutes using a biofeedback machine. "Not only did it help learning about relaxing, but I cured a back problem I had had for about eight years. I got more and more sold on SAGE. I wake up in the morning and see the world as it really is. It's quiet, and you can go over the things you've learned. This is another asset. As for awareness, I'll never be the same. No one ever had a chance at age 70 to live a new life as I have."

Frances Burch, 67, another of the original dozen, found that SAGE opened her to possibilities she had never considered before. "I've seen people in this group change their physical and mental outlook. They're more open and responsive. Their lives are more exciting and they have more possibilities and choices. I feel better physically myself, but it took a long time to convince me that the deep breathing exercises were helpful. I've always been very factual, literal, and skeptical, but I've seen things go on here that are amazing—self-healing."

"I think the most important thing to me is that I'm 68 years old, and probably for the first time in my life, I've experienced real joy in my association with people," said Mac.

"My father was a Presbyterian minister and quite an old fogy, an old-timer. He was a fine man, but he was against dancing, playing cards, and having fun in general. So I truly was an old man most of my life. I wanted to look good. I was taught, 'What will the neighbors think?' so I didn't do what I wanted to do. I did what I thought people would want me to do, but I've gotten over that. I began having fun, enjoying myself, and feeling free to do what Mac would like to do instead of what the neighbors would like me to do. It's a real joy, and I'm grateful."

"Two things," said Ellie Karbach. "One is purely physical. We love each other. We touch, we hug, we do all the things that I've long since almost forgotten except with my family, and, see, this has unbelievable value for an individual. The other thing is that I think somehow or other the whole world is my new world. It's new in the sense of energy, of producing, of meeting friends on a new level. My family is so excited about it. It's almost too much, and yet it's very real. I do honestly feel cosmic."

Working with SAGE has had direct benefits for the teachers as well as the students. Ken Dychtwald told us that he has been more student than teacher while working with these older people. His experience with SAGE has led him to completely reexamine his own values and beliefs about life and death. "I had always believed that to live a 'full life,' one had to live so many years . . . had to tick off so many minutes on the clock. It didn't matter how these years were spent in determining whether or not a life had been full. If Uncle Fred dies at age 93, everyone would probably comment on what a full life he had lived even if he had spent 92 of those years in a state of depression and stagnation. If cousin Johnny, on the other hand, was hit by a car after having lived ten of the most thrilling, creative years you could imagine, it's no doubt that folks would comment on how Johnny never got to live at all. It might very well be that Johnny experienced ten times as much of this stuff we call life as did old Uncle Fred."

Perhaps SAGE's most important contribution has been in giving people, young and old, a chance to develop a new perspective on aging. A project which began in the spirit of "Hey this looks like fun. Let's try jumping up and down or whatever seems appropriate," has blossomed into a new vision of old age's rich potential. *While the subject of death has been repulsive and terrifying to our culture in general, it has hung over older people like a heavy pall, condemning them to a half life while they wait to die.* SAGE seems to be changing that attitude. One group member said that she had begun to look at death "like birth." Another, in her seventies, said, "I look on death as another stage in the adventure." The possibility of positive dying, like that of positive living, is intrinsic in SAGE's work, and as the circle of its influence widens, which it is bound to do given the need for its services and the enthusiasm and direction of its members, we should begin to see a visible transformation in social attitudes about old age. *The positive values of living to an old age and dying consciously have been forgotten in our culture for decades.* It is interesting to watch the ripples SAGE is stirring and to feel the influence and very valuable wisdom of the elders emerging among us again. In a very real way, aging is finally coming of age in America.

If you would like to find out more about SAGE, you can

contact them at Claremont Office Park, 41 Tunnel Road, Berkeley, Calif. 94705. SAGE has made three good video tape documentaries, which are available for rental at a fee of $25 each. The first, running fifty-two minutes, is titled "A New Image of Age." The second, running twenty-five minutes, is titled, "Deep Breathing: Show Me How You Breathe and I'll Tell You How You Live." The third, just being completed (at the time this article was printed), is titled "The SAGE Project: The Coming of Age."

18

The Yoga of Dying Consciously

Death seems not so strange
When one considers night
And all the loveliness there is
When day is gone—
Knowing the brilliance of a burning sun
You'd never know that stars are near
Or that a moon could be—
Or, knowing all the scurry of a busy day,
Suspect that night's deep rest is on its way—
But facing toward a shining sunset sky
And seeing stars and night slip into place—
We would not hold the day with one regret
    that it must go—
We only know that it is right
    that it is so.

—Ruth Brace

Life is full of little unknowns. We never really know for sure what is going to happen from one day to the next, or even from moment to moment. There is always the possibility of the unexpected. Many of us spend our entire lives resisting and denying this fact of life. We want a guarantee that life is going to proceed exactly such-and-such a way. We want to be *sure* of what the next day is going to be like, and we try to predict what is going to happen. Not facing these fears we may have of the little unknowns of life is a major factor in exaggerating the fear of the biggest unknown—death.

Who can say where the body ends and mind begins? Where does the mind end and the spirit begin? It seems that they cannot be divided, as they are all interrelated.

Yogic philosophy teaches that the body is a temporary house for the spirit. The same Power which gave us our body will one day take it away. Though the body is subject to sickness, age, decay, and death, perhaps there is some "essence" within us that remains unaffected.

Recently the problems of the aged and dying have been openly exposed after being tucked away in hospitals, nursing homes, and funeral parlors in what has rightly been called a "conspiracy of silence."

The dying person is preparing, whether he consciously acknowledges it or not, for the confrontation of a totally new, unknown experience.

The only event which we can predict with absolute certainty is that one day we shall have to die, yet it is the one event about which the majority of people refuse to think until forced to do so by the loss of a relative or friend or the realization of the imminence of their own death. It is among the commonest experiences upon the planet; yet we keep the thought of it well out of our consciousness; with the result that when the time comes we are caught unawares and unprepared and unable to do more than reluctantly acquiesce in what, in reality, is a great adventure. . . . (*There Is Only Life,* by Norman Gregor, Sundial House, Nevill Court, Twinbridge Wells, Kent, England.)

The Shanti Project

An area in which yoga and medicine are bridging each other is that of death and dying. In the experience of death the flow of consciousness into a new dimension can be eased by the presence and support of a person whose sensitivity and attunement to the significance of dying (and living) have been enhanced through such disciplines as meditation and yoga.

The actual transitional phase of dying is being increasingly recognized as a nonmedical, natural life process that should occur in a homelike, supportive environment with a person or people present who have the capacity of relating to a human being in transition.

The Shanti Project (Shanti is Sanskrit for "peace") is a training program that prepares volunteers and health-team professionals to be supportive friends to the dying. By merging Eastern, yogic approaches to life with the technological backup of the West (both are needed), a much smoother and trauma-free transition can be possible for the dying.

The Yoga of Serving the Dying

Charles A. Garfield, Ph.D., founder of the Shanti Project, writes in an article, "The Developing Yoga of Dying Consciously" (*Yoga Journal,* September-October, 1975):

Knowledge of death is a universal and uniquely human experience. As conscious beings we are each bound to the realization that "All my loved ones—and I, too—must die." Most of us, however, rarely confront this undeniable reality in an authentic manner. Sharing a culture that tends to deny and camouflage death and dying, we are usually ill-prepared for death—and only vaguely aware that we do not have all the time in this world to live our lives.

Social change in the western world has made illness and death increasingly the responsibility of institutions outside the family—hospitals, nursing homes, and funeral homes. The latest statistics indicate that more than 75% of the present population of the United States will die in hospitals or nursing homes. This means that three out of four of us, in the last days of our lives, will be resocialized to some degree in what has been called a "frighteningly alien terminal subculture."

A very definite shift has taken place in the statistical frequencies of death: a shift toward death from chronic disease. This change, in conjunction with the increased sophistication of therapeutic measures capable of prolonging life, has lengthened the average amount of time that elapses between the onset of a fatal illness and the termination of life. The majority of terminal patients are still faced with the dim picture described by Aldous Huxley as "increasing pain, increasing anxiety, increasing morphine, increasing addiction, increasing demandingness, with the ultimate disintegration of personality and a loss of the opportunity to die with dignity."

While recent findings have publicized the sometimes isolated circumstances under which many die in the hospital context—and hence have started a trend toward self-examination of terminal care on the part of many hospital staffs—there is no systematic provision in the educational processes of professionals for confronting one's own attitudes about death. We often encounter death for the first time with little or no preparation for the emotional impact this event will have upon us.

Several years ago, when I started clinical work with the dying, I became aware that hospital personnel experienced as much fear and avoidance about dying as did the dying themselves. Many physicians and nurses, culturally defined as healers, related to their patients on a bio-medical basis alone. Death is seen as a defeat, a failure, an intruder; it is an adversary in the scientific quest for immortality. Nurses, who often have the most frequent contact with the dying, are often not aware of their own feelings, and frequently avoid any sort of emotional sharing and psychological support of their patients. Psychologists, psychiatrists, and social workers, using general models of mental health intervention, can hide behind their theoretical schemes and psychodiagnostic categories, rather than attempting to interact on a more human and authentic level. There are frequent stories of the alienation of pain, both psychological and physiological, about the abandonment of the dying by family members, of the confusion by nursing and mental health staff, and of the seeming conspiracy of silence often constructed around the dying person.

For reasons more personal than professional, I saw my work with the dying differently; first I had much to learn from my patients. At times I was the student, they the teacher. Once the social mask was abandoned, and the burden of a social image dropped, what was left was two human beings attempting to understand what is often the most perplexing event in all of human experience.

As my work with the dying evolved, there were overwhelming numbers of requests, both from terminal patients and their families, to help with the emotionally demanding aspects of the illness. In addition, I received many requests from hospital staff personnel, especially nursing and mental health staffs, for training experience in working effectively (compassionately) with the dying. It became clear that cultural aversion to the natural conclusion of the life cycle has prevented people from understanding on a personal level what dying and working with the dying are about.

It is vital to remember that we are dealing not with a professional issue but a human one. To pretend that death and dying are processes and events relevant only to those who work in hospital contexts is a gross error. It is helpful to clearly and compassionately realize that we will all be facing "terminal status" and to evaluate and reevaluate our lives in terms of this understanding.

The Shanti Project is a San Francisco Bay Area-based volunteer counseling service for people and their families facing life-threatening illness. The expressed intention is to help train individuals, both professionals and lay people, to provide emotional support to the dying. All volunteers are comfortable and skilled in relating to the dying and their families and believe that this time can be a potentially powerful opportunity for growth and resolution.

Shanti has found that to work effectively with the dying requires a heightened consciousness of death-related feelings, fantasies, thoughts, and actions. The project is exploring the entire sequence of events and emotional and cognitive experiences encountered by both the dying person and the helper, from the initial realization of illness to the actual moment of death.

For further information about the Shanti Project write:

Shanti Project, 1137 Colusa Avenue, Berkeley, Calif. 94707.

Charles Garfield is the coauthor of *Consciousness: East and West* (Harper & Row, 1976) and editor of *Rediscovery of the Body* (Dell, 1977) and *Psychosocial Care of the Dying Patient* (in preparation).

Further Suggested Reading

Light on Yoga, by B.K.S. Iyengar. Schocken Books, 200 Madison Avenue, New York, N.Y. 10016. Paper $4.95. George Allen & Unwin Ltd., London. Cloth.

> Although this book often appears overwhelming for the beginner because of the exact attention to detail and the vast number of asanas that are described, I recommend it highly to the serious student of yoga—beginner or advanced, young or old. It contains 602 photographs, which make it probably the most complete and authoritative work on yoga available in the world today. It is a book that the continuing student of yoga can read and reread over and over, each time learning something new. I especially recommend the Introduction for its clear, beautiful explanation of the eight "limbs" or stages of yoga.

Autobiography of a Yogi, by Paramahansa Yogananda. Self-Realization Fellowship, Publishers, 380 San Rafael Avenue, Los Angeles, Calif. 90065. Paper $1.95. Cloth also available.

> This profound, fascinating account of the life of an authentic Hindu yogi explains with scientific clarity the subtle but definite laws by which yogis perform miracles and attain self-mastery. Colorful chapters are devoted to Yogananda's encounters with saints, masters, and other unforgettable people—Babaji, a two thousand-year-old yogi, Luther Burbank, Sri Yukteswar (his master), and Gandhi.

Yoga Is for You, by Sue Luby. Prentice-Hall, Inc. Englewood Cliffs, N.J. 07632. Paper $2.95.

> Recommended for its clear instruction and photographs of Hatha Yoga, and its reasonable, practical selection of asanas. I only wish the model were not wearing ballet slippers! Otherwise it is a fine book for beginners.

How to Get Well, by Paavo Airola. Health Plus Publishers, P.O. Box 22001, Phoenix, Ariz. 85028. $8.95.

> This is a practical manual on the most common ailments—and what you can do about them—by a world-famous authority on nutrition and natural healing.

Touch for Health, by John F. Thie and Mary Marks. De-Vorss & Company, 1642 Lincoln Blvd., Santa Monica, Calif. 90404. $8.95.

> A practical guide to natural health, using acupuncture, touch, and massage to improve postural balance and reduce physical and mental pain and tension.

Handbook of Natural Remedies for Common Ailments, by Linda Clark. The Devin-Adair Company, 143 Sound Beach Ave., Old Greenwich, Conn. 06870. $9.95.

> This is a useful and sensible book reporting on all aspects of natural methods of treating diseases.

Seeing with the Mind's Eye—The History, Techniques and Uses of Visualization, by Mike Samuels and Nancy Samuels. Random House, 201 E. 50th St., New York, N.Y. 10022. Paper $9.95.

> Visualization—the creation of mental images—is beautifully and extensively presented in this remarkable book, not only as a healing of mind/body technique, but as it affects all the varied aspects of our daily lives. The authors discuss visualization techniques, how to use them to clarify personal goals, and how visualization relates to your life attitudes.

Diet, Sex and Yoga and *Yoga, Science of the Self,* by Marcia Moore and Mark Douglas. Arcane Publications, Box A, York, Maine 03909.

> The first is a particularly inspiring book on the yoga of health. The second covers the whole spectrum of yoga and explains its deeper aspects.

Yoga Journal, 1627 Tenth Avenue, San Francisco, Calif. 94122. $6.00 for one year's subscription.

A bimonthly publication of the California Yoga Teachers Association. Popular and special interest articles on all aspects of yoga, interviews with the world's leading yoga masters, reports on the latest findings in yoga research, new insight on the practice and teaching of yoga.

Formula for Long Life Ends at 168

Shirali Mislimov's formula for a long, happy life was an easy one—a slow pace, clear air, natural food, a kind heart, and work.

His formula was a good one. It kept him going 168 years, making him one of the world's oldest persons.

A peasant, Shirali Mislimov died in his bed in the mountain village of Barzavu (Caucasus, Russia) where he had lived all his life.

In recent years before his death each birthday was an opportunity for the craggy-faced, bearded peasant to tell reporters his philosophy of life:

"I was never in a hurry in my life, and I'm in no hurry to die now.

"There are two sources of long life. One is a gift of nature, and it is the pure air and clean water of the mountains, the fruit of the earth, peace, rest, the soft warm climate of the highlands.

"The second source is people. He lives long who bears no jealousy of others, whose heart harbors no malice or anger, who sings a lot and cries a little, who rises and retires with the sun, who likes to work and who knows how to rest."

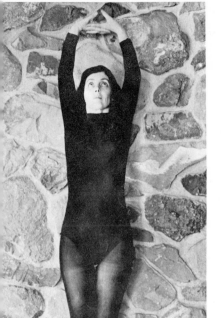

te 1. **Spinal Stretch**

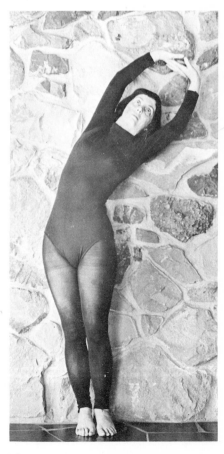

Plate 2. **Side to Side Stretch**

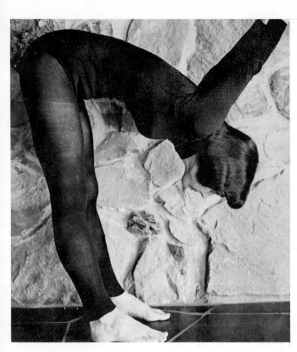

Plate 3. **Instant Energize**

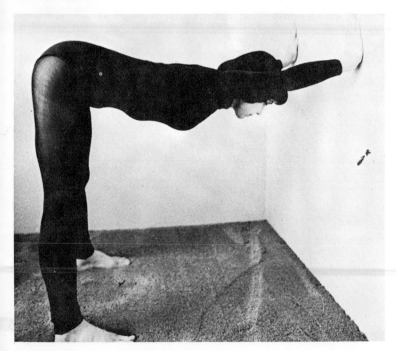

Plate 4. **Back Lengthening**

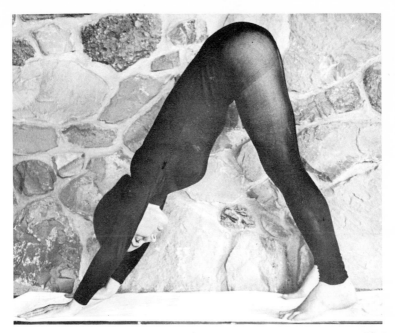

Plate 5. **Downward Facing Dog**

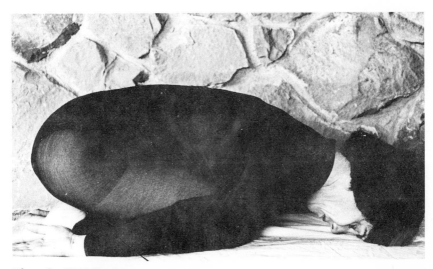

Plate 6. **Child's Pose**

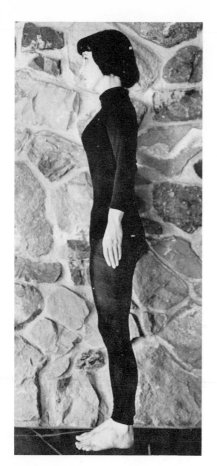

Plate 7. **Mountain Pose**

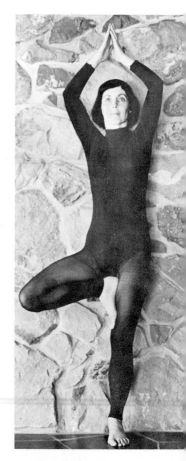

Plate 8. **The Tree**

Plate 9. **Triangle Pose**

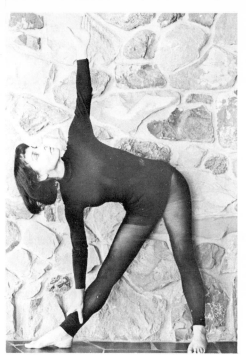

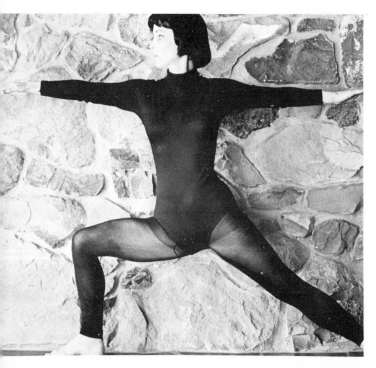

Plate 10. **The "Hero"**

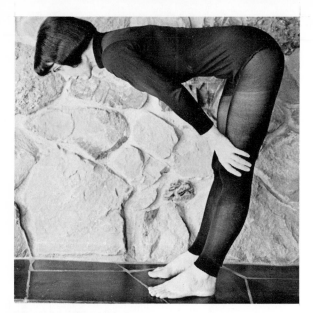

Plate 11. **Standing Forward Bend**

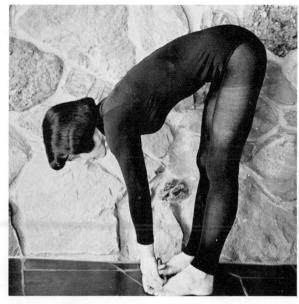

Plate 12. **Big Toe**

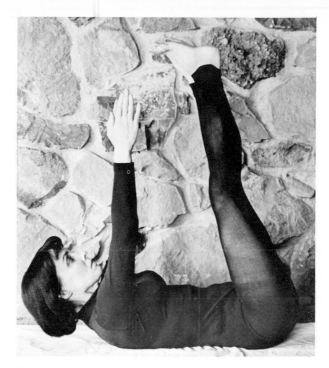

Plate 13. **Upward Extended Hand Foot**

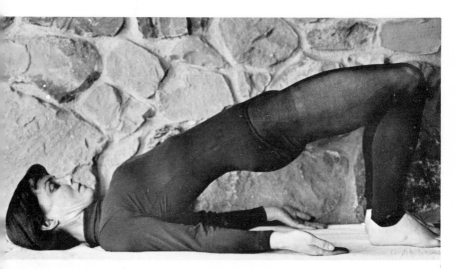

Plate 14. **Bridge Pose**

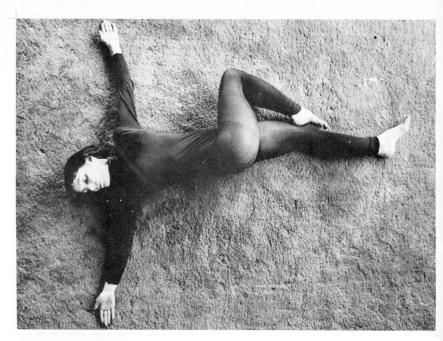

Plate 15. **On-the-Back Twist**

Plate 16. **The Stick Pose**

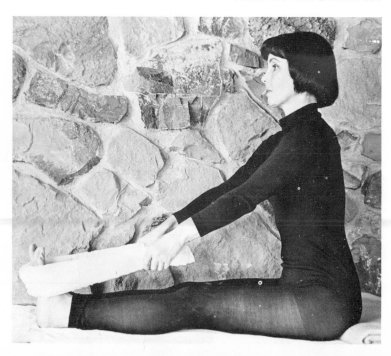

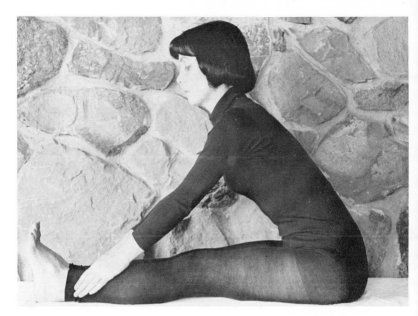

Plate 17. **Basic Full Forward Bend**

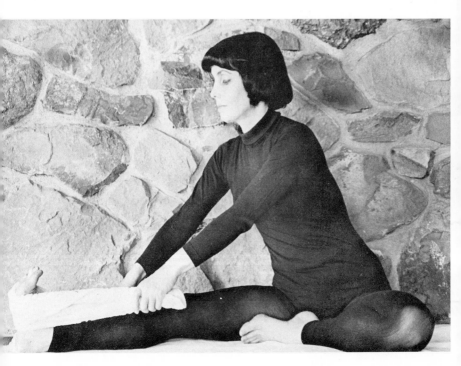

ate 18. **Head to Knee Pose**

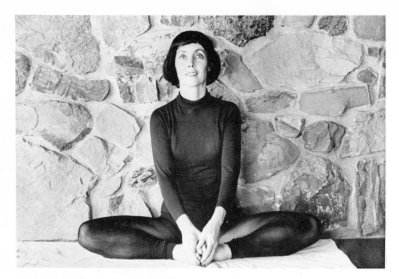

Plate 19. **Bound Angle Pose**

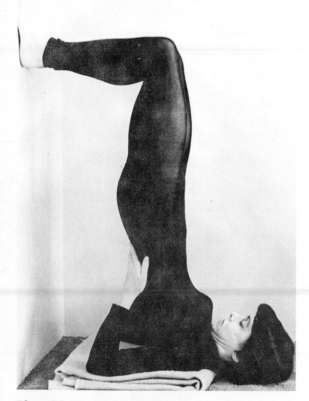

Plate 20. **Supported Shoulder Stand**

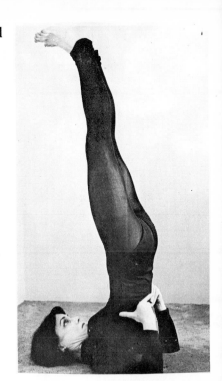

te 21. Shoulder Stand away from wall

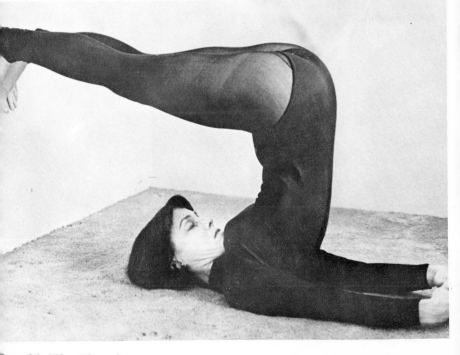

late 22. The Plough

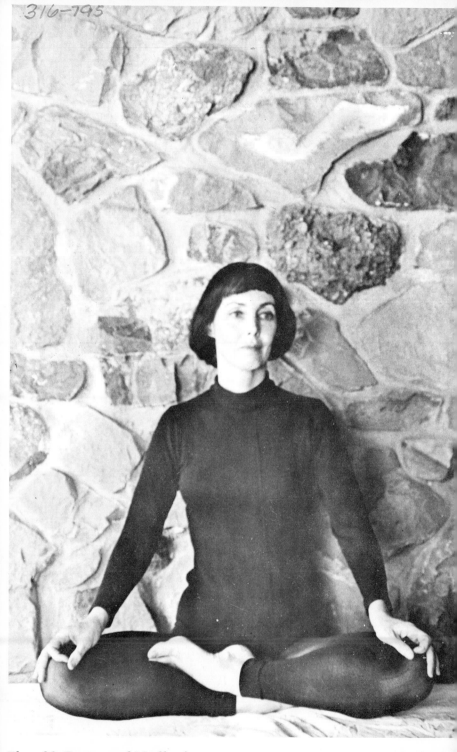

Plate 23. **Posture of Meditation**